A Review of the Scientific Literature As It Pertains to Gulf War Illnesses

VOLUME 1

INFECTIOUS DISEASES

Lee H. Hilborne
Beatrice Alexandra Golomb

Prepared for the Office of the Secretary of Defense

National Defense Research Institute

RAND

Veterans of the Persian Gulf War report a variety of physical and psychological symptoms, some of which remain unexplained. In an effort to determine the extent to which these symptoms may be related to Gulf War service and to develop policies to better deal with health risks in future deployments, the Secretary of Defense designated a special assistant to oversee all Department of Defense (DoD) efforts related to the illnesses of Gulf War veterans. The Office of the Special Assistant for Gulf War Illnesses (OSAGWI) is charged to do everything possible to understand and explain the illnesses, to inform veterans and the public of its progress and findings, and to recommend changes in DoD policies and procedures to minimize such problems in the future.

This literature review, one of eight commissioned by the Special Assistant to the Deputy Secretary of Defense for Gulf War Illnesses, examines the existing scientific literature on what is known about the health effects of infectious diseases that may have affected service members who served in Operations Desert Shield and Desert Storm. The eight RAND reviews are intended to complement efforts by the DoD and other federal agencies as they attempt to understand the full range of health implications of service in that conflict.

The other seven RAND literature reviews deal with chemical and biological warfare agents, depleted uranium, oil well fires, pesticides, pyridostigmine bromide, immunizations, and stress. These represent plausible causes of some of the illnesses Gulf War veterans have reported.

These reviews are intended principally to summarize the scientific literature on the known health effects of given exposures to these risk factors. Where available evidence permits, the other seven reviews also summarize what is known about the range of actual exposures in the Gulf and assess the plausibility of the risk factor at hand as a cause of illness. Statements related to the Gulf War experience should be regarded as suggestive rather than definitive, for more research on health effects and exposures remains to be completed before definitive statements can be made. Recommendations for additional research where appropriate are included.

These reviews are limited to literature published or accepted for publication in peer-reviewed journals, books, government publications, and conference proceedings. Unpublished information was occasionally used, but only to develop hypotheses. This review covers literature published before the spring of 1999 but in some cases includes additional references primarily as a result of the peer-review process.

This work is sponsored by the Office of the Special Assistant and was carried out jointly by RAND Health's Center for Military Health Policy Research and the Forces and Resources Policy Center of the National Defense Research Institute. The latter is a federally funded research and development center sponsored by the Office of the Secretary of Defense, the Joint Staff, the unified commands, and the defense agencies.

CONTENTS

FIGURE

TABLES

Following the Gulf War, some veterans of that conflict began reporting a variety of health conditions and other symptoms, some of which remain unexplained. The Department of Defense (DoD), as part of its effort to inquire into possible causes of these illnesses, has commissioned various studies of the scientific literature about potential or contributing causes of illnesses in Gulf War veterans.[1] This document represents one such study. It focuses on infectious diseases with the goal of presenting current medical knowledge regarding these diseases, irrespective of the specific issues surrounding the Gulf War. When appropriate, it interprets whether a particular infectious disease or related condition is likely to explain symptoms experienced by those who served in the Gulf War.

Infectious diseases have been extensively studied and their identification, diagnosis, and treatment are generally well understood. Therefore, this study does not consider all infectious diseases. Rather, it focuses on known or plausible ones—those that were actually diagnosed in people who served in the Gulf War or that are known either to exist in the Persian Gulf area or to produce symptoms similar to those experienced by Gulf War veterans. A complete review of the scientific literature, even as it pertains to the discussed infectious diseases, is beyond the scope of this volume.

An early study by the Centers for Disease Control and Prevention showed three types of symptoms as being about three times more prevalent among those who had served in the Gulf War: chronic fatigue, joint and muscle pain, and neurocognitive symptoms. However, the symptoms described were not unique to service in the Persian Gulf War.

---

[1]Throughout this report the term "Gulf War illnesses" is intended to refer generally to symptoms experienced by veterans who served in the Gulf War, irrespective of whether those symptoms are explained or unexplained.

After the review of the scientific literature about infectious diseases, we make the following observations:

- Of the known infectious diseases (i.e., known to have infected veterans or known to be present in the area of the conflict), none seems likely to cause the undiagnosed illnesses in Gulf War veterans.

- That said, the patterns of infectious diseases have some similarities to some cases of undiagnosed illnesses among Gulf War veterans. Therefore, we cannot entirely rule out some unknown infectious disease as a possible cause of illness for some individuals.

- At present, most commonly recognized infectious diseases have been ruled out as a major factor among ill Gulf War veterans. One theory that continues to merit investigation concerns the role of *Mycoplasma* infection as a cause. More testing is currently under way to evaluate the relationship between *Mycoplasma* infection and illness in Gulf War veterans.

INFECTIOUS DISEASES

A case can be made both for and against infectious diseases as a cause of the illnesses among Gulf War veterans. The argument for an infectious cause includes the belief that symptoms reported by Gulf War veterans represent an epidemic among a group of people with a common exposure, in this case service in the Middle East during the war. History bolsters this interpretation. Typically, some time passes before a cause is identified for an observed set of symptoms. AIDS is a case in point. In that case, several years passed after the observation of a set of symptoms before a virus and diagnostic test were identified. Furthermore, some of the infectious diseases diagnosed among Gulf War participants, most notably *Leishmania*, produce some symptoms similar to those described by Gulf War veterans.

However, some factors weigh in against infectious disease as a cause. For example, the veterans do not have a common, measurable sign, such as a fever, abnormal laboratory test, or anatomic lesion (e.g., sores, rash). Although some veterans present anatomic lesions, the lack of a consistent set of signs and symptoms makes it difficult to conclude that a single infectious disease could be the cause.

INFECTIOUS DISEASES AMONG GULF WAR VETERANS

During the earliest stages of deployment when the weather was extremely hot, acute diarrheal disease was the major infectious disease problem (Hyams et al., 1995). The most commonly identified enterpathogens were multidrug-resistant enterotoxigenic *Escherichia coli* (ETEC) and *Shigella sonnei*. There were no laboratory-confirmed cases of cholera, typhoid fever, amoebic dysentery, or giardiasis. Viral gastroenteritis became a problem after the weather became cooler in December 1990. Acute upper respiratory infections were also prevalent, especially during periods of crowded travel and billeting (Hyams et al., 1995).

In this deployment, there were no documented cases of sandfly fever, and outbreaks of febrile illness consistent with insect-borne infections were not reported (Richards et al., 1993). There was one confirmed case of West Nile fever, seven cases of malaria among U.S. troops who went into southern Iraq, and three cases of Q fever. Brucellosis was not diagnosed among western troops, and viral hepatitis was an infrequent problem. One chronic infectious disease that has been linked to service in the Middle East was viscerotropic leishmaniasis. This sandfly-transmitted infection has been diagnosed in 12 U.S. veterans but not in other coalition personnel (Magill et al., 1993). Viscerotropic leishmaniasis is a comparatively mild form of systemic leishmanial infection caused by *Leishmania tropica*, a eukaryotic parasite that typically produces cutaneous disease. In addition, 20 U.S. Gulf War veterans have been diagnosed with cutaneous leishmaniasis caused by *L. major* infection (Kreutzer et al., 1993).

OTHER DISEASES

Several diseases known to exist in and around the Kuwaiti Theater of Operations were not identified in any of the veterans. These include sandfly fever (phlebotomus fever), dengue fever, typhus, and brucellosis. Other infections also were considered as possibly related, including mycoplasmosis, tuberculosis, anthrax, and botulism. The latter two were considered because they are biological warfare agents.

LEISHMANIA

Leishmania is a vector-borne parasite transmitted in Southwest Asia by the sandfly, *Phlebotomus papatasi*. It is of interest to the study of the illnesses among Gulf War veterans because it exists in the Kuwaiti Theater of Operations, causes some of the same symptoms observed in the illnesses among Gulf War veterans, and has been found in some of the veterans. Although different species of *Leishmania* look the same under a microscope, they have different effects on their hosts. Two types of syndromes—cutaneous and visceral leishmaniasis—are of particular interest because they exist in the area, and both have been diagnosed in veterans. The cutaneous form appears two to eight weeks following infection, although some cases have been reported as long as a year later. It manifests itself as ulcers that form at the site of the bite. Twenty cases of this type of leishmaniasis were diagnosed. Visceral leishmaniasis involves multiple organs in the body, can be quite virulent, and can result in death. The type experienced by the Gulf War veterans appears to be a milder form, termed viscerotropic leishmaniasis, and 12 cases have been diagnosed.

BIOLOGICAL WARFARE AGENTS

Coalition troops feared, with some justification, that Iraq might use biological weapons against them. The two most likely candidates were anthrax and botulinum toxin. Fortunately, both are well understood and diagnosis, treatment, and prevention strategies exist for each. Both agents have severe, life-threatening symptoms, and neither is known to have a chronic state. Thus, if these agents were used against coalition troops, we would have expected multiple individuals to become symptomatic shortly after exposure. Low-level exposures do not appear likely.

MYCOPLASMA

Mycoplasmas are the smallest free-living microorganisms, and cause disease in plants, animals, and humans. One strain has been reported in a number of veterans who have the symptoms of the Gulf War illnesses. A technique called nucleoprotein gene tracking has been developed to detect the bacteria in patients, and a rigorous study has been designed and is under way to validate this technique and compare it to a more established technique, namely, the polymerase chain reaction. Meanwhile, several sources have reported high rates of *Mycoplasma* in ill Gulf War veterans using genetic techniques. Tests assessing antibody production against *Mycoplasma* have not produced these high rates, but many people may not generate antibodies to this organism if infected, reducing the sensitivity of antibody techniques for detecting *Mycoplasma* infection.

UNIDENTIFIED INFECTIONS

A final possibility is that a previously unidentified infectious disease is causing illnesses among Gulf War veterans. There is no positive evidence to suggest that this is the case; however, it cannot be ruled out. Some of the routine tools for identifying differences between those with and without illnesses among Gulf War veterans are not available because too much time has passed. Other techniques, for example, screening pre- and postwar blood samples, have been tried on available samples but to date have yielded no positive results. Other sophisticated techniques, such as DNA or genetic analysis, are possible.

ACKNOWLEDGMENTS

We wish to thank the many individuals who contributed to our understanding of the issues presented in this document. Special thanks are due to Dr. Michael Wilson (University of Colorado) and Dr. William C. Reeves (Centers for Disease Control and Prevention, Atlanta, Georgia) for their contributions and review of the early drafts of this manuscript. We thank Dr. Joel Baseman, Dr. Darryl See, Dr. Harold Watson, Dr. Barry Cole, Dr. Joe Tulley, Dr. Chuck Engel, Dr. Shyh-Ching Lo, and Dr. Garth Nicolson for helpful discussions pertaining to the *Mycoplasma* chapter. We also thank Dr. Donald Henderson (Johns Hopkins School of Public Health) and Dr. Robert Chen (CDC).

Chapter One

INTRODUCTION

BACKGROUND

Troops based in the Arabian Gulf during World War II experienced high morbidity rates from infections. Because of this, coalition troops in the Gulf War were expected to face considerable risk of sandfly fever, malaria, diarrheal disease, and cutaneous leishmaniasis (Quin, 1982). To monitor these expected infections, the U.S. military established a diagnostic laboratory in Saudi Arabia to collect extensive surveillance data.[1] However, history did not repeat itself, and these diseases did not affect a significant portion of those serving in the Gulf regions.

A combination of factors was probably responsible for the resulting low rates of serious infectious disease (Hyams et al., 1995). Rapid medical care was available for acute diarrheal and respiratory infections, reducing morbidity. Also, extensive preventive medicine efforts, including vaccinations, immune serum globulin for hepatitis A prophylaxis, the use of insect repellents, camp hygiene, and monitoring of food and water supplies, helped reduce the transmission of infectious diseases.

Two chance factors may have played an even greater role in reducing infectious disease morbidity: the time of year when most troops were deployed (the cooler winter months) and the location of the deployment (the barren desert) (Hyams et al., 1995). Cold weather reduced the risk of insect-borne diseases at the height of the buildup, as did deployment of most troops away from areas where arthropod vectors and mammal hosts are most plentiful. In comparison, World War II troops were stationed throughout the year and were more likely to camp in oases, river areas of southern Iraq, and urban locations where infectious diseases are a greater threat (Quin, 1982).

---

[1]GulfLINK.osd.mil Medical Surveillance during Operations Desert Shield/Desert Storm, November 6, 1997 (www.gulflink.osd.mil/nfl).

PURPOSE

Still, numerous Gulf War veterans have reported a range of symptoms, some of which are similar to those caused by diseases prevalent in the Gulf region. Therefore, infectious diseases merit consideration as a potential cause of these symptoms.

The scope of infectious diseases is massive, encompassing both the hundreds of known infectious organisms and also the diseases and syndromes they cause. The topic has generated volumes of scientific work and is reviewed well elsewhere. We do not attempt to deal with all infectious diseases in this report. Rather, we focus on known or plausible infectious diseases associated with the Persian Gulf. By known diseases we mean those that were identified in those who served in the Persian Gulf during the Gulf War. Plausible diseases include those known to exist in the area and, more broadly, those whose signs and symptoms are similar to those experienced by Gulf War veterans. We present a short summary of etiology, diagnosis, and treatment and also review the literature related to infectious diseases that were unusual to or of great concern in the Gulf (e.g., mycoplasma disease and leishmaniasis).

ORGANIZATION OF THIS DOCUMENT

This chapter provides a general overview of infectious diseases, describing what we know about them and how they are known to behave. It discusses infectious diseases known to have occurred among those who served in the Gulf War and infectious agents common to the Gulf region. The second chapter briefly discusses infectious disease epidemiology (the study of diseases in groups of people as opposed to studies of diseases in individuals).

Following chapters discuss specific infectious diseases by category of infectious organism, including bacterial (Chapters Three and Four), viral (Chapter Five), and parasitic (Chapter Six) infections. Chapter Seven discusses anthrax and botulinum toxin—the two biological agents thought to be most likely to be used by the Iraqis against the troops in the Gulf War. Chapter Eight presents current methods employed to search for new and emerging diseases and the final chapter gives conclusions and recommendations. An appendix contains additional information about *Mycoplasma*.

OVERVIEW OF WHAT WE KNOW ABOUT DISEASES

Despite scientific advances over the years, medical science has not identified every possible disease or every possible interaction between infectious organisms and humans (Lederberg, 1997). For example, not too many years ago, a constellation of clinical findings (e.g., organic pathology) that we now know as the Acquired Immune Deficiency Syndrome (AIDS), was identified in a group of patients. Patients presented with a number of different findings, although all related to the function of the immune system, ranging from unusual infectious diseases to rare cancers. Only later was the Human Immunodeficiency Virus (HIV) identified as the infectious agent responsible for these various manifestations. Similarly, for many years a causative agent for gastritis remained unidentified. Recently, *Helicobacter pylori* was identified as a common causative and treatable agent. The main difference between these conditions and those of Gulf War illnesses is that symptoms, without measurable clinical findings, are much less definable in the latter.

As the above discussion shows, there is a natural scientific evolution to what we know about infectious diseases. Typically, some unusual combination of findings results in further study, sometimes taking years, that ultimately identifies a cause, sometimes an infectious disease. Given the symptoms of Gulf War illnesses, it is not surprising that an infectious etiology has been considered among the potential causes. Some of the symptoms are found in patients infected with known agents. However, some of the findings suggest that this explanation, while certainly possible, is unlikely.

The Iowa Persian Gulf Study Group (1997) conducted the first population-based epidemiological study to evaluate the health consequences of the Gulf War. The 3,695 subjects who participated in this study were selected from a larger population of almost 29,000 military personnel who listed Iowa as their home. Furthermore, they were specifically selected to represent individuals from all four branches of the military, including both regular military personnel and National Guard and reservists. The interviews for the study were conducted by telephone, resulting in a high rate of participation. Seventy-six percent of the eligible study subjects completed the detailed interviews and the response rate was 91 percent among persons contacted by telephone. The study included a carefully selected comparison group of military personnel who were not deployed to the Persian Gulf but who served during the time of the Gulf War. The Iowa study found that military personnel serving in the Gulf War were more likely than those who did not to report symptoms suggestive of cognitive dysfunction, depression, chronic fatigue, post-traumatic stress disorder, and respiratory illness (asthma and bronchitis). The conditions identified in the Iowa study appear to have had a measurable effect on the functional activity and daily lives of Gulf War veterans and only minimal differences were observed between National Guard or reserve troops and regular military personnel.

Likewise, the Centers for Disease Control and Prevention (CDC) studied Air Force personnel, and that study significantly contributed to our understanding of the health consequences of the Gulf War (Fukuda et al., 1998). That study or-

ganized symptoms reported by Air Force Gulf War veterans into a case definition, characterized clinical features, and evaluated risk factors. The cross-sec-
tional questionnaire was sent to 3,723 currently active volunteers from four Air
Force populations. Clinical evaluations were performed on 158 Gulf War veterans from one unit, irrespective of health status. A case was defined as having
one or more chronic symptoms from at least two of three categories (fatigue,
mood-cognition, and musculoskeletal) and was further characterized as mild-
to-moderate or severe depending the severity of the symptoms. The prevalence
of mild-to-moderate and severe cases was 39 percent and 6 percent, respectively, among 1,155 Gulf War veterans compared to 14 percent and 0.7 percent
among 2,520 nondeployed veterans. Fifty-nine (37 percent) clinically evaluated
Gulf War veterans were noncases, 86 (54 percent) were mild-to-moderate cases,
and 13 (8 percent) were severe cases. The key observation of the study was that
Air Force Gulf War veterans were significantly more likely to meet certain criteria for severe and mild-to-moderate illness than were nondeployed personnel
(Fukuda et al., 1998). There was no association between the chronic multisymptom illness and risk factors specific to combat in the Gulf War (month or
season of deployment, duration of deployment, duties in the Gulf War, direct
participation in combat, or locality of Gulf War service). The finding that 15
percent of nondeployed veterans also met illness criteria was equally important
and suggests that multisymptom illness observed in this population is not
unique (although less frequent) to Gulf War service. The clinical evaluation
component of the study found that neither mild-to-moderate nor severe cases
were associated with clinically significant physical examination or routine laboratory abnormalities. However, Gulf War veterans classified as having mild-to-
moderate and severe illness (cases) had a significant decrease in functioning
and well-being compared with noncases.

COMMON ILLNESSES IN GULF WAR VETERANS

Table 1.1 shows the distribution of complaints expressed by veterans.[2] When
those with symptoms were medically evaluated, a specific diagnosis was made
for 77 percent. Among veterans with symptoms who did not receive a specific
diagnosis, a characteristic physical sign or laboratory abnormality was not observed.

Similar data are available for individuals who remained on active duty. They
have been encouraged to refer themselves for care. Data on these individuals
are maintained as part of the Department of Defense (DoD) Comprehensive
Clinical Evaluation Program (CCEP) (1996). Table 1.2 describes the common

---

[2]Veterans in the Persian Gulf Health Registry with complaint data available.

Table 1.1

Common Complaints of Gulf War Veterans
(Persial Gulf Health Registry with complaint data available)

Complaints	% Women n = 4,919	% Men n = 42,705
Fatigue	23	21
Headache	23	18
Skin rash	18	19
Muscle, joint pain	15	17
Memory loss and other general symptoms	14	14
Shortness of breath	8	8
Sleep disturbances	5	6
Abdominal pain	4	3
Other skin symptoms	4	3
Diarrhea and other gastrointestinal symptoms	4	5

SOURCE: Institute of Medicine (1996).

Table 1.2

Common Complaints of Individuals Who Served in the Gulf War
(n = 18,075 CCEP Participants)

Symptoms	Any Complaint (%)	Chief Complaint (%)
Joint pain	49	11
Fatigue	47	10
Headache	39	7
Memory problems	34	4
Sleep disturbances	32	2
Skin rash	31	7
Difficulty concentrating	27	<1
Depression	23	1
Muscle pain	21	1
Diarrhea	18	2
Shortness of breath	18	3
Abdominal pain	17	3

SOURCE: Institute of Medicine (1996).

complaints expressed by the 20,000 CCEP registrants as of April 1996 (IOM, 1996; DoD, 1996). All complaints are recorded, including the chief complaint (i.e., the main reason for seeking care).

The symptoms and complaints listed in Tables 1.1 and 1.2 are real. In fact, most of us have experienced one or more of them. It is important to understand, therefore, whether Gulf War veterans experience these symptoms and complaints more than they would have had they not served in the Gulf War. If the rate of these symptoms and complaints is higher than that of the general population, we must then consider whether the increase is or might be related to infectious diseases.

The following discussion places the roles of infectious diseases, and the spectrum of illness experienced by Gulf War veterans, into three general categories:

1. Infectious diseases known to have occurred among Gulf War troops.

2. Infectious diseases known to exist in the Persian Gulf region but not diagnosed in any of our troops.

3. Other infectious diseases considered as possible causes of Gulf War illnesses.

INFECTIOUS DISEASES IN GULF WAR TROOPS

The most complete evaluation of the effect of infectious diseases on Gulf War troops covers cases reported during Operations Desert Shield and Desert Storm (August 1990 to March 1991) and any cases up to early 1994 that were reported and attributed to service during that period (Hyams et al., 1995).

Gastrointestinal Diseases

Gastrointestinal (GI) complaints were the most frequent symptom among deployed U.S. troops (Hyams et al., 1991). Most who experienced transient symptoms found that they resolved after a few days. Although present throughout the deployment, GI problems were most frequent during the early days (August and September 1990), probably because fresh produce was obtained locally (from Mediterranean and Asian sources). In October 1990, once exposure to fresh produce was stopped, the rate of GI complaints declined dramatically. By November/December, the rate dropped to about 0.5–1.0 percent seeking treatment per week, similar to what is experienced among civilians in a community health care setting. Table 1.3 lists the gastrointestinal pathogens identified among symptomatic Gulf War troops.

Respiratory Diseases

Respiratory diseases were common among troops stationed in the Middle East. In an epidemiological study of 2,598 male ground troops, 34 percent reported a sore throat, 43 percent a cough, and 15 percent a persistent runny nose (Richards et al., 1993). Not surprisingly, as in civilian environments, symptoms were treated without confirming a specific cause. Specific studies to look for a cause for disease were undertaken in only 68 individuals (Table 1.4).

Other Diseases

Other diseases known to occur in the Middle East were experienced by a small number of individuals (Table 1.5).

Table 1.3

Gastrointestinal Infections Identified Among Individuals Serving in the Gulf War

Infectious Organism	Type	Number
Escherichia coli	Bacterial	
Toxin producing		125
Invasive		3
Shigella species	Bacterial	113
Salmonella	Bacterial	7
Campylobacter	Bacterial	2
Norwalk virus	Viral	9

SOURCE: Hyams et al. (1991).

Table 1.4

Respiratory Pathogens Identified Among Individuals Serving in the Gulf War

Infectious Organism	Type	Number
Streptococcus pyogenes	Bacterial	3
Neisseria meningitidis	Bacterial	4
Streptococcus pneumoniae	Bacterial	1
Haemophilus influenzae	Bacterial	1
Mycoplasma pneumoniae	Bacterial	1
Influenza (types A and B)	Viral	3
Adenovirus	Viral	1

SOURCE: Richards et al. (1993).

Table 1.5

Other Infections Identified Among Individuals Serving in the Gulf War

Infectious Organism	Type	Number
Leishmania tropica (viscerotropic)	Protozoa	12
Leishmania major (cutaneous)	Protozoa	20
Plasmodium vivax (malaria)	Protozoa	7
Coxiella burnetii (Q fever)	Rickettsia	3
West Nile fever	Virus	1

SOURCE: Hyams et al. (1995).

INFECTIOUS DISEASES IN THE PERSIAN GULF BUT NOT IDENTIFIED IN GULF WAR TROOPS

Experience with previous wars in the Middle East led military and civilian experts to predict that the number of patients who might experience infectious diseases native to the Persian Gulf would be higher than was actually experienced. Several specific infections were known to exist in and around the Persian Gulf region, yet they were not identified among U.S. troops. These infectious diseases include those listed in Table 1.6.

Table 1.6

**Infections Common in the Persian Gulf
But Not Diagnosed Among Individuals
Serving in the Gulf War**

Infectious Disease	Type
Phlebotomus (sandfly) fever	Virus
Dengue fever	Virus
Sindbis	Virus
Rift Valley fever	Virus
Brucellosis	Bacteria
Spotted fever diseases	Rickettsia
Typhus diseases	Rickettsia
Schistosomiasis	Trematode
Echinococcosis	Tapeworm

SOURCE: Hyams et al. (1995).

OTHER INFECTIOUS DISEASES CONSIDERED

Several other infectious diseases have been considered as possibly related to Gulf War illnesses,[3] although they are not specific to the region in which United States troops were deployed. Specific diseases considered are listed in Table 1.7.

---

[3]As noted in the summary, in this volume the term Gulf War illnesses is used to indicate the range of undiagnosed illnesses experienced by veterans of the Gulf War. We use the term to refer to the sum of conditions experienced by veterans of the Gulf War; we do not imply that there is or is not one disease.

Table 1.7

Other Infections Possibly Related to Gulf War Illnesses

Infectious Organism	Type
Epstein-Barr virus	Virus
Mycoplasma fermentans	Bacteria
Mycoplasma penetrans	Bacteria
Mycobacterium tuberculosis	Mycobacteria
Bacillus anthracis[a]	Bacteria
Clostridium perfringens[a]	Bacteria
Clostridium botulinum[a]	Bacteria

[a]Considered because they are biological warfare agents (see Chapter Seven).

Chapter Two

INFECTIOUS DISEASES AS A POSSIBLE CAUSE OF GULF WAR ILLNESSES

Several concepts and diseases are discussed in the chapters that follow. But first, it is useful to consider why, in the search for answers about unexplained illnesses and findings in Gulf War Veterans, it is reasonable to consider an infectious origin and why an infectious etiology does not seem likely. Arguments for and against an infectious etiology are presented and discussed.

REASONS TO CONSIDER AN INFECTIOUS ETIOLOGY

Epidemiologic Relationship

Epidemiology is the study of diseases in a population or group of people. Most of us are familiar with epidemics—for example, an influenza (flu) epidemic occurs when there is an increase in the number of cases above a baseline. An epidemic may be of short duration (e.g., food poisoning) or of long duration (e.g., cancer), but the common element is that a specific disease emerges with increased frequency over what would otherwise be expected. A second premise assumes that the increased incidence of disease follows a unique exposure or exposures.

Concern about Gulf War illnesses exists because many believe that the unexplained symptoms in Gulf War veterans might represent a constellation of findings in increased frequency among our Gulf War veterans. Like the flu or cancer, then, the unexplained illnesses represent an increase relative to the baseline (the epidemic) in a group of individuals with a common exposure (service in the Middle East during the Gulf War).

History of Infectious Diseases

Chapter One reviewed some concepts surrounding the natural evolution of diseases that have subsequently been shown to have an infectious cause. Medical science today knows more about causes of illnesses than it ever has before. But clearly we do not know all the answers. Before a specific cause is found, diseases and syndromes are described clinically; that is, they are characterized by how patients describe their illness to their physicians, the findings that the physician observes during a physical examination, or the presence of abnormalities in the results of diagnostic studies (e.g., x-rays, blood and urine tests). With further study, including epidemiologic studies, possible causes are identified. Often, but not always, a common cause is identified for a constellation of clinical findings.

The natural history of most infectious diseases is such that some time passes before an infectious cause is identified. In fact, some infectious diseases, such as cholera, were recognized before the causative organism was identified. In the case of cholera, public health measures reduced the risk of gastrointestinal problems including diarrhea, dehydration, and death long before the causative bacteria, *Vibrio cholerae*, was isolated. More recently, the AIDS epidemic was recognized by a group of clinical and epidemiologic characteristics two years before the specific virus was identified. Similarly, only recently has *Helicobacter pylori* been identified as one cause of gastritis (inflammation of the stomach).

Some Infectious Diseases Were Identified

Infectious diseases, although not nearly as common as in past military deployments, were diagnosed during and after the Gulf War. The most notable is leishmaniasis because some of the Gulf War illness symptoms are consistent with the way some patients with *Leishmania* actually feel. It is also clear that we still have much to learn about this infection and the way it interacts with our bodies. Other infections, including hepatitis and tuberculosis, also can and do manifest as chronic diseases.

REASONS TO DISMISS AN INFECTIOUS ETIOLOGY

Koch's Postulates

Robert Koch, a physician and microbiologist in the late 1800s and early 1900s, provided a set of criteria that established the experimental evidence required to support the relationship between a specific microorganism and a disease. The criteria have expanded over the years, but the basic principles still serve as the basis for establishing a relationship between an organism and a disease. Koch's postulates state:

1. The microorganism must be observed in every case of the disease;

2. The microorganism must be isolated and grown in pure culture;

3. The pure culture must, when inoculated into a susceptible animal, reproduce the disease; and

4. The microorganism must be observed in, and recovered from, the experimentally diseased animal.

These guidelines provide a useful framework for the discussion that immediately follows. To date, Koch's postulates have not been satisfied among those with Gulf War illnesses. However, Koch's postulates are often not completely satisfied in illness. Completely satisfying Koch's postulates provides strong evidence for a causal relationship; but inability to satisfy all postulates does not exclude a causal link between the organism and the disease.

A Missing Specific Finding

In one important way, unexplained Gulf War illnesses differ from some of the diseases just discussed. In the case of AIDS, researchers and epidemiologists described specific clinical findings that could be verified by laboratory tests, x-rays, and clinical examination. There were also lifestyle risk factors that were highly associated with the disease. Physicians readily identified gastritis in patients harboring *H. pylori*, even though the infectious agent was not initially related to that observation. In contrast, despite attempts to demonstrate reproducible objective findings, no specific clinical findings or laboratory abnormalities have been observed in those identified with unexplained Gulf War illnesses. Usually, if there is a common thread to a specific disease, there will be common objective findings. Most infectious diseases are characterized by findings such as fever, abnormal laboratory tests, organ derangement, or specific outcomes such as recovery, paralysis, and death. For example, patients with hepatitis have jaundice (yellow skin) and abnormal liver tests; those with pneumonia have increased white blood cell counts and abnormal chest x-rays, and those with severe emphysema (a noninfectious example) have abnormal x-rays, lung tests, and physical findings. Because the reported findings in ailing Gulf War veterans with unexplained symptoms are few and not consistent from veteran to veteran, the lack of objective and consistent findings makes it difficult to conclude there is a single common pathological process or cause.

Some Evidence Does Not Fit

The Experience of Coalition Countries. U.S. forces worked closely with military forces from other countries. If the cause of illnesses in some Gulf War veterans is infectious, then it is spread to victims through some common exposure. If the exposure is unique to the Gulf region, then one would expect that those serving from other countries would experience illnesses at roughly the same rate as U.S. troops. However, efforts to identify similar illnesses in coalition troops have not been confirmed to the same degree (i.e., at the same rate) as in U.S. Gulf War veterans. Some individuals from the United Kingdom report similar illnesses but in numbers considerably fewer than have been observed in U.S. veterans (DoD, 1996; Defense Science Board, 1994). However, because of different definitions of "disease" in different countries and different motivations among those who seek care for a given problem, it is difficult to draw firm conclusions regarding prevalence of similar findings in other countries.

Family Studies. As of December 1995, there were 332 spouses and 191 (119 of whom had a diagnosis other than "healthy") children who were registered as part of the DoD CCEP. Because the CCEP is a clinical program with self-reporting rather than a population-based program, it is not possible to draw conclusions about the true prevalence of disease among military spouses and children. However, the number of children and spouses reporting illnesses in this registry does not exceed what might be expected in a population the size of the Persian Gulf deployment (697,000 troops). If considerable Gulf War illness was caused by an infectious agent that could be transmitted directly between Gulf War veterans in the Middle East, we might expect more direct person-to-person transmission among family members who would therefore have illnesses similar to those included among the Gulf War illnesses. It is possible, however, that even if person-to-person transmissible diseases did exist, their period of infectivity (contagious period) may have passed by the time they returned home.

Chapter Three

BACTERIAL DISEASES (MYCOPLASMA)

One theory suggests that illnesses in Gulf War veterans may result from infection with *Mycoplasma*—bacteria-like microorganisms that are the smallest free-living microorganisms. This chapter considers the *Mycoplasma* theory. It first discusses briefly the *Mycoplasma* species, including how they affect healthy persons and those with compromised immune systems. It then discusses hypotheses regarding how Gulf War veterans might have been infected with *Mycoplasma* and relates evidence for and against these hypotheses. It recounts the debate surrounding testing methods for *Mycoplasma* infection and provides preliminary data regarding response to antibiotic treatment of ill Gulf War veterans who test positive for *Mycoplasma*.

BACKGROUND ON MYCOPLASMAS

Mycoplasmas belong to the class Mollicutes. They are the smallest organisms capable of self-replication in cell-free media. (Lo, 1992). Like bacteria, they contain no nucleus but do contain DNA and RNA; however, unlike most bacteria, they have no cell wall (Lo, 1992; Marty, 1993). They cause serious disease in many animal species (as well as plants), where they may affect multiple organ systems or cause chronic disease. *Mycoplasmas* are often difficult to detect and to eradicate. They may elude the immune system, and they may alter it (inducing appearance of a lymphokine profile, or a set of signaling cells produced by those immune cells termed lymphocytes, that favors activation of B-lymphocytes that are involved in antibody production), possibly precipitating autoimmune disease (Baseman et al., 1996; Baseman and Tully, 1997). A *Mycoplasma* has been proposed as the most likely ancestor of the animal mitochondrion (Pollack, 1997; Karlin and Campbell, 1994). Mitochondria are elements within the cell that serve as the principal source of energy to the cell. *Mycoplasma* proteins are sufficiently similar to animal proteins (Baseman, 1996) that either the body's immune system may not recognize *Mycoplasmas* as foreign or they may cause the body to make autoantibodies that attack the host animal and produce autoimmune disease.

Mycoplasma and Disease in Those with Dysfunctional Immune Systems

Mycoplasmas are commonly opportunistic organisms (pathogens) that cause illness principally in those whose immune systems are not fully functioning (e.g., persons with AIDS, genetic immune deficiency syndromes, or receiving chemotherapy for cancer or organ transplantation) (Lo, 1992). They have also been postulated to serve as cofactors in the development of AIDS in HIV-infected persons (Lo, 1992) (see below).

Mycoplasma and Disease in Those with Normal Immune Function

Mycoplasma pneumoniae is the most common cause of pneumonia in normal young adults. *Mycoplasma genitalium* is considered a cause of nongonococcal urethritis (NGU, a sexually transmitted disease) in humans. Its presence in men with urethritis (inflammation of the urethra—the canal from the bladder that allows discharge of urine to outside the body—causing pain and discharge from the penis) is independent of the presence of the more commonly recognized urethritis-causing agent *Chlamydia trachomatis*. Using a technique called polymerase chain reaction (PCR), in which genetic material is amplified to improve organism detection, *M. genitalium* was found in urethral samples from 23 percent of 103 men with signs or symptoms of NGU but in only 6 percent of 53 men without NGU ($p < .006$) (Marty, 1993). Response to treatment with the antibiotic doxycycline was at least as satisfactory in resolving symptoms in those with confirmed *M. genitalium* as in those with *C. trachomatis*, further supporting the role of *Mycoplasma* in causing the symptoms (doxycycline is effective against the *Mycoplasma*). *M. genitalium* has been implicated in pelvic inflammatory disease (PID), a serious consequence of sexually transmitted infection in women where the infection travels into the pelvis possibly resulting in infertility. Approximately 25 percent of infertile women have antibodies to *M. genitalium* (Marty, 1993), and this infection is increasingly considered a possible cause of male and female infertility. *M. genitalium* is also found in the respiratory tract and may cause disease in the respiratory tract independent of any genital disease (Baseman and Tully, 1997). *M. hominis* is also associated with PID and increased risk of preterm delivery. Fulminant respiratory distress syndrome and failure of multiple organ systems have been described with *M fermentans* in immunocompetent individuals (Lo, 1992). Congenital infection (infection at birth in infants who acquired infection in utero) with *Ureaplasma urealyticum*, also a *Mycoplasma*, is associated with central nervous system damage, chronic lung disease of prematurity, neonatal bacteremia, pneumonia, meningitis, premature spontaneous labor and delivery, and possibly a condition termed "hydrops fetalis" (Marty, 1993) involving abnormal accumulation of fluid in fetal tissues.

MYCOPLASMA IN GULF WAR VETERANS

It has been proposed that *Mycoplasma* infection may have contributed to illnesses in Gulf War veterans, possibly through contaminated anthrax vaccines. Supporting this theory, two investigators have reported high rates of positive tests for *Mycoplasma* in ill Gulf War veterans (in one instance, using a new technique called nucleoprotein gene tracking that remains to be externally validated; and in the other, using PCR.[1] One reports that many of those who tested positive responded favorably to antibiotic treatment, often with resolution of long-standing severe symptoms.

Some members of the scientific community have criticized this theory, raising four objections. First, no significantly increased rates of conversion to *Mycoplasma*-antibody-positive status, from pre- to postdeployment, were found using stored blood from Gulf War veterans enrolled in a Gulf War health registry compared with those not so enrolled. Second, the newly devised test is itself new and unproven. Third, *Mycoplasma* could not plausibly grow in anthrax vaccine (one postulated mechanism of transmission). Finally, they observe that no controlled trials of treatment have been published (although such a trial is currently under way) (Duerksen, 2000).

Evidence supporting a connection between illness in Gulf War veterans and *Mycoplasma* derives almost exclusively from non-peer-reviewed sources. Such evidence cannot prove that *Mycoplasma* is a cause of illness in Gulf War veterans. However, this preliminary evidence provides a strong case for additional research into this putative mechanism.

Several distinct subhypotheses are implicit in the *Mycoplasma* hypothesis as articulated by its author, Garth Nicolson. These subhypotheses may be examined for their independent merits. Elimination or confirmation of one subhypothesis does not imply elimination or confirmation of the others. Furthermore, each subhypotheses engenders a set of questions. Table 3.1 presents each subhypothesis and the related questions.

EVALUATING ELEMENTS OF THE MYCOPLASMA HYPOTHESIS

For each set of questions, the next section reviews available information.

---

[1]Recent news reports confirm that an ongoing federally funded study has also found similar high rates of positive tests for *Mycoplasma* in ill Gulf War veterans (Duerksen, 2000).

Table 3.1

Subhypotheses and Related Questions

Subhypothesis	Related Question
Anthrax vaccine given to Gulf War veterans may have been contaminated with *Mycoplasma*	**Origin**: What is the evidence favoring and opposing anthrax vaccine as a source of *Mycoplasma* agents? What are other postulated origins of *Mycoplasma* as a cause of disease in Gulf War veterans?
Nucleoprotein gene tracking is a reliable and valid testing method for *Mycoplasma*	**Testing**: It has been reported that nucleoprotein gene tracking and Forensic PCR more reliably detect *Mycoplasma* infections than traditional PCR, and therefore reliably distinguish patients who carry, or are infected with, *Mycoplasma* from those who do not or are not. Others challenge the plausibility of these reports, questioning whether these tests are reproducible and if they really are superior to traditional PCR.
Mycoplasma is a plausible source of illness in ill Gulf War veterans	**Theoretical plausibility**: Irrespective of concerns about the origin of the *Mycoplasma* agent, is present knowledge of *Mycoplasma* characteristics theoretically consistent with the possibility that *Mycoplasma* could produce disease such as that seen in Gulf War veterans?
Data support the presence of *Mycoplasma* in ill Gulf War veterans	**Evidence**: What are the data regarding presence of, or infection with, *Mycoplasma* in ill Gulf War veterans?
Ill Gulf War veterans who test positive for *Mycoplasma* (using nucleoprotein gene tracking or PCR) respond to antibiotics	**Treatment**: Irrespective of whether *Mycoplasma* is the etiology, does treatment with stated antibiotics lead to symptom abatement or resolution in ill Gulf War veterans who do and do not test positive for *Mycoplasma*?

Origin

The theory regarding an anthrax vaccine origin for *Mycoplasma*-induced illness is speculative. The theory's author first considered *Mycoplasma* as a cause of illness in a subject who became chronically ill after volunteering for military medical experiments involving vaccinations and who tested positive for *Mycoplasma*. Subsequently, Nicolson saw ill Gulf War veterans in whom *Mycoplasma* was also detected, using methods he devised (Nicolson and Nicolson, 1997) (see below).[2]

The possibility of accidental contamination as a source of *Mycoplasma* in anthrax vaccines can be scrutinized in light of current understanding of *Mycoplasma*. *Mycoplasma* frequently contaminates mammalian (or, more generally, eukaryotic) cell lines and tissue cultures (Baseman and Tully, 1997), such

---

[2]G. Nicolson, letter, 1997.

as those in which viral vaccines are grown. For this reason, *Mycoplasmas* are tested for at the start of and at the end of the viral vaccine production process.

The anthrax vaccine (the main "new" vaccine given in the Gulf War) is made in a sterile synthetic medium that would be presumed unfavorable to *Mycoplasma*. *Mycoplasmas* are fastidious organisms difficult to culture even from diseased tissue (Lo, 1992). They have complex nutritional requirements and depend on external supplies of biosynthetic precursors, including amino acids, nucleotides, fatty acids, and sterols (Baseman and Tully, 1997). Moreover, many tissue and blood components inhibit *Mycoplasma* growth (Lo, 1992). Experts suggest that if the *Mycoplasma* could survive, it would quickly be "outcompeted" by the much faster growing bacteria and die out. Moreover, both anthrax (AX) and botulinum toxoid (BT) vaccines (the BT vaccine being the other new vaccine) contain formaldehyde as a "cross-linker" in BT vaccine and as a stabilizer in AX vaccine. BT vaccine also contains thimerosol, a mercury compound, as a preservative and AX vaccine has "phemerol," or benzethonium chloride, as a preservative. These preservatives would be "expected" (experts believe) to kill *Mycoplasma* unless very high *Mycoplasma* levels were introduced (Hardegree et al., 1997). At present no peer-reviewed studies have been found that studied the levels of the preservatives required to kill *Mycoplasma*.

A few have argued that *Mycoplasma* infection resulting from accidental *Mycoplasma* contamination of anthrax vaccines is unlikely or impossible (Food and Drug Administration (FDA), 1996). The DoD performed tests for *Mycoplasma* on anthrax vaccine batches and state that it found no contamination. A formal scientific-style report of this work, including full methods and results, has not yet been published in the peer-reviewed literature, nor has this finding been reproduced by DoD-independent scientists.

Nicolson and Nicolson (1997) reported that two ill British Gulf War veterans tested positive for *Mycoplasma*. Since the British anthrax vaccine differed from the U.S. vaccine in many respects, and was manufactured independently, this would seem to reduce the likelihood of contamination in the manufacturing process as a source of *Mycoplasma* infection in Gulf War veterans.

However, many sources of *Mycoplasma* contamination are possible (Baseman and Tully, 1997); therefore, the true likelihood of *Mycoplasma* contamination of vaccines is difficult to gauge. Both the FDA and the military have viewed *Mycoplasma* contamination of anthrax vaccines as very unlikely, based on information such as that described above (FDA, 1996). They have judged the possibility as low enough to merit no additional follow-up. However, the only reference identified in which anthrax vaccine was *tested* for *Mycoplasma did* report *Mycoplasma* contamination. *Mycoplasma* was cultured from Iraqi (local) anthrax vaccine (Alshawe and Alkhateeb, 1987) although no Iraqi vaccine was used by the United States, and vaccine production methods in Iraq may differ substantially from production methods in the United States. (Direct information regarding Iraqi production methods is lacking.)

There is no direct or epidemiological evidence connecting *Mycoplasma* to the anthrax vaccine or to any other vaccines received by Gulf War veterans. However, the theory of mycoplasmal illness does not depend on the contamination of anthrax (or other) vaccines as a source; and vaccines are not the only possible source by which *Mycoplasma* infection might have emerged.

Other sources of pathogenic *Mycoplasma* have been postulated. For instance, there are suggestions that *Mycoplasma* may be endemic in the Middle East in sand or water, that the Iraqis may have used it as a biological weapon, or that it was dispersed as "blow-back" after their biological weapon stores were destroyed (Nicolson and Nicolson, 1996; Moehringer, 1997; Offley, 1996). Because of the difficulty growing *Mycoplasma*, many view *Mycoplasma* as an unlikely biological warfare agent. Some suggest that pathogenicity may have been enhanced by immune dysfunction resulting from other multiple vaccinations or other exposures or from breach of the blood-brain barrier (Nicolson and Nicolson, 1997), such as may have occurred with multiple chemical exposures or stress (see the companion report on pyridostigmine bromide (Golomb, 1999)). These theories do not involve a direct vaccine provenance for the *Mycoplasma*. Additionally, evidence suggests that immune system changes may occur as a consequence of exposure to acetylcholinesterase inhibitors (see Golomb, 1999, and the companion report on pesticides (Cecchine et al., 1999)), so that it is possible that individuals with these or other exposures may have enhanced susceptibility to infection with intracellular bacteria such as *Mycoplasma*.[3]

---

[3]Regarding the first of these hypotheses, that *Mycoplasma* is endemic in areas where Gulf War troops were deployed, discussions with Saudi, Kuwaiti, and Egyptian medical personnel indicate that symptoms of the type described in U.S. Gulf War veterans were not common in Saudi, Kuwaiti, or Egyptian troops or civilians. No local disease with these symptoms has been described. Thus, endemic *Mycoplasma* disease with these symptoms appears unlikely unless native immunity is present or illness reporting is poor. However, mycoplasmal disease cannot be absolutely excluded. Cultural differences may influence illness reporting. For example, cancers in these populations frequently present with quite advanced, highly visible disease. Local physicians may discount illness for which objective findings have not been isolated, complicating exclusion of such illness. Indigenous populations could have relative immunity to similar illness either through genetic selection or advantages produced by early exposure.

Possibly consistent with these theories is the suggestion by U.S. medical personnel in Saudi Arabia that symptoms similar to those seen in Gulf War veterans may be common in Americans stationed in that area after, and possibly before, the Gulf War (E. McClure, personal communication to Beatrice Golomb, 1997; M. Kamel, personal communication to Beatrice Golomb, 1997). However, quantitative information on such reports of symptoms is not available. In one observational study of all encounters in one year in a Saudi Arabian primary care practice, 33.5 percent had chronic problems. Musculoskeletal and digestive disorders, among the most prominent symptoms in ill Gulf War veterans, accounted for 38 percent and 24 percent of encounters, respectively (Al-

Testing of Veterans for Mycoplasma

Historically, testing for *Mycoplasma* has been problematic.[4] As mentioned, *Mycoplasmas* are fastidious and difficult to grow from diseased tissue. They may not provoke a marked antibody response, so that serological testing to detect antibodies to *Mycoplasma* is unreliable. The *Mycoplasma* particles, which occur in different forms (pleomorphic) and lack a tell-tale cell wall, are difficult to distinguish from fragments of extracellular cytoplasm or cell organelles released from degenerating cells.[5] A validated, readily available diagnostic test for *M. fermentans incognitus* has not been available for routine use.

Different investigators, using distinct testing methods, report dramatically different prevalence of *Mycoplasma* infection in ill Gulf War veterans (Table 3.2). Specifically, higher prevalence rates of *Mycoplasma* have been reported in ill Gulf War veterans than in controls by one investigator who employed nucleoprotein gene tracking and forensic PCR. Higher rates have also been reported in a small sample of ill Gulf War veterans than in a large sample of controls by another investigator using traditional PCR. A third investigator found no statistically significant increase in conversion to antibody positivity in Gulf War veterans who applied to a Gulf War registry compared with those who had not, and overall rates of positivity for *M. fermentans* were low using antibody tests. (As mentioned above, recent preliminary results from an ongoing large study support the possibility of high rates of positivity in ill Persian Gulf War veterans.)

Two factors may be responsible for discrepancies in the findings of the investigators, namely, testing differences and subject selection. Regarding testing methods, PCR and possibly nucleoprotein gene tracking may be more sensitive, whereas serological testing is insensitive and may miss true cases. As noted above, serological testing may not be reliable, because a significant antibody response may not be produced in response to *Mycoplasma*.[6]

Indeed, each testing method has been criticized. Skepticism regarding nucleoprotein gene tracking has been voiced by some who doubt that a technique (nucleoprotein gene tracking) that fails to involve amplification could be more sensitive than one that does (traditional PCR). Nucleoprotein gene tracking is a

---

Shammari and Nass, 1996). But the data collection and presentation strategy do not permit determination of whether any of these subjects had combinations of symptoms like those reported by ill Gulf War veterans.

[4] S. Lo, personal communication to Beatrice Golomb (1997).

[5] S. Lo, personal communication to Beatrice Golomb (1997).

[6] S. Lo, personal communication to Beatrice Golomb (1997).

Table 3.2

Mycoplasma Test Results in Gulf War Veterans and Controls

Investigator	% Gulf War Veterans Testing Positive	% Controls Testing Positive	Test	# Cases/ # Controls Tested	Gulf War Sample
Lo (1993)[a]	3[b]	NA	Antibody—not sensitive	27/0	Registry participants
Lo (converters) (1994)[a]	2.6[c]	1.3	Antibody—not sensitive	151/151	Registry participants
Nicolson, Nicolson, and Nasralla (1998)	45	5	Nucleoprotein gene tracking[d]— not validated	170/41	Ill Gulf War veterans
See (1997)[e]	70	7	PCR	20/>100	Ill Gulf War veterans

[a]As reported in Ribas (1996).

[b]Three positive for *M. fermentans* or *M. penetrans*.

[c]*M. fermentans.*

[d]Also forensic PCR.

[e]D. See, personal communication to Beatrice Golomb (1997).

new technique that has not yet been tested by outside groups, and reproducibility and validity remain to be demonstrated (testing is under way). Moreover, some researchers question whether forensic PCR (a PCR strategy developed for use when only small blood samples are available) would be more sensitive than traditional PCR when an adequate blood sample is available.[7] However, with traditional PCR, unless care is taken, the genetic material to be amplified may fail to be accessed.[8] Forensic PCR and nucleoprotein gene tracking are reportedly designed to help circumvent this problem.[9] Finally, antibody tests, although established, are thought to be insensitive and often fail to detect *Mycoplasma* infection. Other testing factors (e.g., differences in "blinding" of patient status during analysis of test results) could in principle contribute to the testing differences. In this scenario, reports of the high rates of *Mycoplasma* positivity in ill Gulf War veterans may be spurious results of bias in categorization.

The second factor that may help explain discrepancies in study results is differences in subject selection. The investigators who reported high rates of

---

[7]S. Lo, personal communication to Beatrice Golomb (1997); H. Watson, personal communication to Beatrice Golomb (1997).

[8]J. Baseman, personal communication to Beatrice Golomb (1997).

[9]G. Nicolson, personal communication to Beatrice Golomb (1997).

Mycoplasma positivity in ill Gulf War veterans may see particularly ill patients or patients whose primary symptoms are loosely consistent with chronic fatigue and fibromyalgia and who may have a different pathogenesis of disease. The investigator who found no difference in *Mycoplasma* prevalence between cases and controls defined as a case any patient enrolled in a Gulf War health registry, and defined as a healthy control any Gulf War veteran not enrolled. Yet many Gulf War veterans who report increased symptoms following the war have not elected to enroll in a Gulf War registry. Moreover, not all veterans enrolled in a registry report illness. "Misclassification bias" of ill and healthy veterans resulting from use of registry data would be expected to produce a bias toward the null,[10] that is, bias that would favor failure to detect a true difference, if there is one.

The reliability of nucleoprotein gene tracking and forensic PCR and their performance compared to traditional PCR are amply amenable to empiric evaluation. A large DoD-funded study is under way to investigate proposed and generally accepted diagnostic techniques for *Mycoplasma* and the validity of various testing techniques, including nucleoprotein gene tracking and forensic PCR.[11] Sixty ill Gulf War veterans (defined as having two of three of the following: six months fatigue, pain in more than one part of the body, and neurocognitive deficits) have been tested using Nicolson's protocol. Of the 60, 30 are individuals not previously tested, 10 are individuals known to be nucleoprotein gene tracking negative, 10 are known to be forensic PCR negative, and 10 are known positive by conventional PCR. Each patient sample is to be tested four times, once by Baseman (University of Texas), once by Lo (Armed Forces Institute of Pathology), and twice by Nicolson (to ensure test-retest reliability). It is expected that preliminary data analysis will be forthcoming in the near future.

Theoretical Compatibility of Mycoplasma Infection with Symptoms in Gulf War Veterans

Setting aside debates regarding the possible origin of alleged *Mycoplasma* infection in ill Gulf War veterans and the debate over testing methods, there is relatively more agreement among experts that a *Mycoplasma* could in principle

---

[10]Provided that the misclassification is "nondifferential."

[11]S. Lo, personal communication to Beatrice Golomb (1997); G. Nicolson, personal communication to Beatrice Golomb (1997); C. Engels, personal communication to Beatrice Golomb and Lee Hilborne (1997).

cause the chronic symptoms seen. However, different levels of enthusiasm exist for this hypothesis.[12]

Mycoplasmas often localize to the joints, and some species produce arthritis in animals (Baseman et al., 1996; Cole and Ward, 1979).[13] *Mycoplasmas* are speculated to produce joint-related symptoms in humans;[14] such symptoms are prominent among Gulf War veterans (Joseph, 1997). Moreover, *Mycoplasmas* may localize to the mucous lining of the mouth, the respiratory tract, and the genital tract. Genital infection is postulated to cause infertility in men and women,[15] and *Mycoplasma* has been proposed as a source of endometritis and prostatitis.[16]

Apropos of *Mycoplasma* as an illness etiology in Gulf War veterans, *Mycoplasma fermentans* has been postulated as a cause of rheumatoid arthritis, although data attempting to confirm a link have been inconsistent.[17] (However, preliminary data reported by Darryl See (personal communication, 1997, chronic fatigue syndrome and rheumatoid arthritis), a published abstract (Huang, See, and Tilles, 1997), and two reports published since this review appear to confirm high rates ofmycoplasma positivity in both chronic fatigue syndrome (Huang, See, and Tilles, 1997; Nasralla, Haier, and Nicolson, 1999), and rheumatoid arthritis (Haier et al., 1999). Nonetheless, recent randomized treatment trials with antibiotics have confirmed a response to long-term (6–12 months) active antibiotic treatment (such as azithromycin or doxycycline, or recently minocycline (O'Dell et al., 1997)) significantly exceeding that of placebo, with arrest of progression of joint erosion and abatement of symptoms.[18] *Mycoplasma* cannot at this point be confirmed to be a cause of rheumatoid arthritis, but antibiotic treatment is effective regardless of the etiology.

Evidence of Mycoplasma in Ill Gulf War Veterans

Sources differ to date in detection of *Mycoplasma* in ill Gulf War veterans, as shown in Table 3.2. In one study *Mycoplasma* species were reported in 45

---

[12]S. Lo, H. Watson, G. Nicolson, C. Engels, J. Tully, personal communication to Beatrice Golomb (1997).

[13]H. Watson, personal communication to Beatrice Golomb (1997).

[14]J. Tully, personal communication to Beatrice Golomb (1997).

[15]J. Tully, personal communication to Beatrice Golomb (1997).

[16]Genital symptoms, particularly painful intercourse in spouses of Gulf War veterans, were a common complaint in an informal review performed of a convenience sample of charts of family members of Gulf War veterans presenting to the San Diego Veterans Administration as part of the Gulf War evaluation.

[17]J. Tully, personal communication to Beatrice Golomb (1997).

[18]J. Tully, personal communication to Beatrice Golomb (1997).

percent of 170 tested Gulf War veterans using a novel testing technique, nucleoprotein gene tracking, that has not yet been evaluated for reproducibility, compared with approximately 5 percent of 41 healthy nonveteran adult controls (Nicolson and Nicolson, 1997). In a second study, the rate of *Mycoplasma fermentans* detection, using serological tests, was not significantly higher in Gulf War veterans who entered a registry than in those who had not, nor was the rate of serological conversion significantly higher. Preliminary data from a third unpublished study (see Tables 3.2 and 3.3) indicate positive tests for *Mycoplasma fermentans* in 70 percent of those ill Gulf War veterans who have been evaluated (14 of 20), compared with approximately 7 percent of "hundreds" of healthy controls (D. See, personal communication, 1997). The prevalence of *Mycoplasma fermentans incognitus* identified by PCR for ill Gulf War veterans is reportedly similar to that detected in patients with chronic fatigue syndrome with immune deficiency markers (CFIDS). Sixty-eight percent of CFIDS patients test positive for *Mycoplasma* (and a similar fraction for herpes-virus 6). Patients with chronic fatigue without immunodeficiency markers have a positivity rate similar to healthy controls. Nicolson and colleagues (1996) observed that symptoms in ill Gulf War veterans are similar to those in patients with CFIDS. Of note, *Mycoplasma* species were identified, using PCR, from the synovial fluid of about 60 percent of patients with rheumatoid arthritis.[19]

Table 3.3

M. Fermentans Incognitus by PCR, Using Primers Specific for a Hairpin Region of M. Incognitus, on Peripheral Blood Mononuclear Cells

Subjects	Published % Mycoplasma Positive	Published # Mycoplasma Positive	Revised % Mycoplasma Positive[a]
Healthy	20	6/30	5–10
Chronic fatigue syndrome without markers			~10
AIDS	40	12/30	40
Rheumatoid arthritis			60–70
Chronic fatigue syndrome with immune deficiency markers	68	57/84	68
Ill Gulf War veterans			70

SOURCES: D. See, personal communication with Beatrice Golomb (1997); Huang et al. (1997).

[a]Current numbers based on "hundreds of cases" for each category, except Gulf War n = 20 (Huang et al., 1997)

---

[19]D. See, personal communication to Beatrice Golomb (1997).

In short, different investigators report markedly different prevalence of *Mycoplasma* in ill Gulf War veterans. These differences may result from differences in testing techniques and/or from differences in subject selection. Because two investigators report a high prevalence of *Mycoplasma* in ill Gulf War veterans and a third (using an insensitive technique and different criteria for case and control subjects) does not, further work should be done to evaluate and to standardize testing techniques, and to determine if high *Mycoplasma* positivity is confirmed in ill Gulf War veterans compared with healthy controls using sensitive, validated testing methods.

Treatment of Veterans with Antibiotics

No controlled trials of antibiotics for illness in Gulf War veterans have been published to date. Nicolson and colleagues (1996) published a case series (uncontrolled) in which improvement of symptoms is reported in Gulf War veterans who were treated with antibiotics for a long time (doxycycline, azithromycin, ciprofloxacin, clarithromycin). There are few reports of success using other treatment strategies. Six-week treatment cycles with antibiotics have been used, reportedly because physicians had little experience with, and showed reluctance to treat with, longer courses of antibiotics. The data from Nicolson and Nicolson (1997) indicate essentially universal (100 percent) relapse after a single six-week course, with successively increasing recovery rates in subsequent cycles (Table 3.4). However, follow-up time after each cycle is not given, and it is possible that apparent "recovery" after later treatment cycles reflects insufficient follow-up time to detect the next "relapse." Indeed the authors of this study speculated that the condition may not be cured but only controlled with antibiotics. *Mycoplasmas*, with their putative deep penetration into the cell (intracellular sightings have been made in eukaryotic cells from infected patients and tissue cultures using electron microscopy and anti-*Mycoplasma* antibodies (Baseman et al., 1995)) and their ability to evade host surveillance systems, are particularly difficult to eradicate. Concern exists that partial treatment may lead to antibiotic resistance.[20] Moreover, *Mycoplasmas* may reside in cells for six months despite antibiotic treatment.[21] Therefore, if *Mycoplasma* is confirmed to be present selectively in ill Gulf War veterans and if treatment trials are undertaken, longer treatment courses may be needed such as those used in successful antibiotic trials for rheumatoid arthritis (six months to a year).

---

[20]S. Lo, personal communication to Beatrice Golomb (1997).

[21]J. Baseman, personal communication to Beatrice Golomb (1997).

Table 3.4

**Recovery of Ill Gulf War Veterans
with Antibiotic Treatment**

# of Six-Week Antibiotic Treatment Cycles Completed	% Relapsing
1	100
2	89
3	73
4	50
5	27
6	19

SOURCE: Nicolson and Nicolson (1997).

Other physicians have also anecdotally reported benefit to ill veterans with antibiotic treatment (Ribas, 1996).[22] Many such veterans and their family members have reported marked resolution of chronic debilitating symptoms with antibiotic treatment.[23] To date, however, no controlled trials have been completed to confirm or refute the benefit of antibiotics. A large-scale, federally funded randomized controlled trial is presently under way and has enrolled all 450 subjects needed at the time of this printing.

CORRELATION WITH GULF WAR ILLNESSES

Data are not available that conclusively support or refute *Mycoplasma* as a source of illness in Gulf War veterans. Factors favoring or consistent with infectious etiology of symptoms in ill Gulf War veterans from an organism such as *Mycoplasma* include variably delayed onset of illness, multiple organ system involvement, chronic symptomatology (*Mycoplasmas* are able to establish covert or overt chronic and persistent infections with concomitant activation of the immune system (Baseman and Tully, 1997)), putative communicability, purported response to antibiotics, and reported (but unsubstantiated and elsewhere contradicted (Asa et al., 2000)) worsening with steroid administration. If antibiotics were confirmed to produce marked attenuation of symptoms in even a portion of seriously ill veterans, this would constitute an important finding, since resolution of symptoms in ill veterans is the goal of greatest importance to these veterans and their families. For this reason, the *Mycoplasma* hypothesis merits serious scrutiny. (Note that symptom resolu-

---

[22]K. Leisure, personal communication to Beatrice Golomb (1997).

[23]Letters to Garth Nicolson from C. Hamden, P. Zalewski (1994); E. Geonetta, B. Harris, L. Millett, L. Roberts, R. Snyder, R. Toth (1996); Burnett and Burnett (n.d.).

tion does not confirm *Mycoplasma* as the etiologic agent; other infections responding to the antibiotic could theoretically be culpable.)

Moreover, if *Mycoplasma* (or other unidentified infectious bacterial disease) is construed as an unlikely source of illness in ill Gulf War veterans, testing is a fortiori important, because veterans are currently seeking treatment with antibiotics. If antibiotic treatment is ineffective, veterans should have the benefit of high-quality data demonstrating lack of efficacy. Because *Mycoplasma* infections are difficult to eradicate and *Mycoplasmas* survive long-term recommended antimicrobial treatment in humans and in tissue cultures (Baseman and Tully, 1997), consideration should be given to a long treatment trial to enhance likelihood of eradication and to minimize development of antibiotic resistance resulting from partial treatment. The postulated intracellular location of the organism and the extreme duration of therapy that led to initial success in rheumatoid arthritis cases might be construed as favoring quite a long duration of therapy, perhaps six months to one year, in a treatment trial. Consideration should be given, during such long-term treatment, to incorporating strategies to maintain intestinal flora and reduce risk of intestinal fungal overgrowth. (As mentioned above, since this report was reviewed and this recommendation generated, a multisite randomized trial of long-term antibiotic versus placebo in ill Gulf War veterans testing positive for *Mycoplasma* has been initiated and is now well under way.)

SUMMARY

Mycoplasma has been postulated as an etiology for illness in Gulf War veterans. Although some have proposed anthrax vaccine contamination, this appears unlikely, because *Mycoplasma* growth requirements may be incompatible with the sterile vaccine medium and the preservatives (formaldehyde and benzethonium chloride) included in the vaccine, although the possibility of vaccine contamination cannot be excluded definitively. Investigators agree that *Mycoplasma* can be responsible for chronic multisystem symptoms. Although investigators disagree on whether ill Gulf War veterans have increased incidence of positive tests for *Mycoplasma*, more sensitive testing methods do appear to show increased rates. Experts agree in principle that *Mycoplasma* could be responsible for chronic symptoms such as those seen in ill Gulf War veterans, although other infections or noninfectious etiologies could be responsible instead or in addition. Definitive studies are currently under way to evaluate testing strategies to detect possible *Mycoplasma* infection.

Table 3.5

Synopses of *Mycoplasma* Studies in Gulf War Veterans

Author	Test System	Results	Considerations	Conclusions
Lo (1993)[a]	Antibodies to *M. fermentans* or *M. penetrans*, *M. genitalium* (27 sera tested)	1 positive for *M. fermentans*, 1 positive for *M. penetrans*, 5 positive for *M. genitalium*	Small sample size, identification of cases and controls problematic, lack of peer review, and methodology relatively insensitive	*M. fermentans* and *M. penetrans* are unlikely to play an etiologic role in Gulf War illness
Lo (1994)[a]	Antibodies to *M. fermentans* or *M. penetrans*, *M. genitalium* (151 cases from CCEP registry with non-CCEP Gulf War veterans as matched controls) using pre- and postdeployment stored sera. Positive antibody confirmed by Western Blot	*M. fermentans*: 10 cases and 10 controls positive pre- and post-deployment; 4 cases and 2 controls seroconverted. Adjusted OR = 2.3 (95% CI 0.4–13.1); *M genitalium*: 56 cases and 56 controls positive pre- and postdeployment; 9 cases, 13 controls seroconverted; adjusted OR = 0.6 (95% CI 0.2–1.7); *M. penetrans*: 1 case and 1 control seroconverted	Not peer-reviewed; CCEP registration not a good classification; methodology relatively insensitive tests; cryopreserved specimens; pre- and postdeployment data provide distinct advantage; sample size may be inadequate because of estimates of positivity in population	No significant association between ELISA/Western Blot positivity for tested *Mycoplasma* species and being a CCEP participant
Nicolson, Nicolson, and Nasralla (1998)	Nucleoprotein gene tracking (NGT) used to test for *Mycoplasma* in ill Gulf War veterans	NGT positive lymphocytes in 45% (76/170) of those with Gulf War illness who "loosely fit clinical criteria for Chronic Fatigue Syndrome with Fibromyalgia"; nondeployed healthy controls positive in less than 5% (2/41)	Cases and controls poorly defined, NGT not yet shown to be reliable or valid, trial is nonrandomized, unblinded	Treated patients recovered following several 6-week cycles and reverted to *Mycoplasma* negative; multiple treatment cycles required for response to treatment
See (1997)[b]	PCR used to test for *Mycoplasma* in ill Gulf War veterans	14/20 (70%) tested positive for *Mycoplasma* genetic material	Unpublished, non-peer-reviewed data, limited sample size; PCR is a sensitive and proven method for detection	Possible high rate of positivity for *Mycoplasma* using PCR

[a]As reported in Ribas (1996).   [b]D. See, personal communication to Beatrice Golomb (1997).   OR = odds ratio.   CI = confidence interval.

Chapter Four

BACTERIAL DISEASES (OTHER THAN MYCOPLASMA)

TYPHOID FEVER

Introduction

Typhoid fever is a life-threatening illness caused by the bacterium *Salmonella typhi*. The infection is common through the world except in the United States, Canada, Australia, Japan, and Western Europe. There are about 400 cases per year in the United States. *S. typhi* colonizes only humans, so spread of the disease requires close contact with an infected individual, either somebody with an active infection or a chronic carrier. The infection is transmitted via the fecal-oral route, and the most common method by which infection is acquired is through consumption of contaminated food and water. Infected individuals have the bacteria in the blood and digestive tract. A small percentage of individuals recover from the acute infection but become carriers and continue to shed the bacteria and therefore remain infectious. The classical case is that of "Typhoid Mary" Mallon who infected many individuals for whom she prepared food as a professional cook.

What Infected Patients Experience

The incubation period for typhoid fever depends on the amount of organism ingested and the immune status of the patient, with a range from a few days to one or two months. Then the patient experiences the insidious onset of a sustained fever with temperatures up to 103°F–104°F accompanied by headache, malaise, anorexia, relative bradycardia (out of proportion to what would be expected with high fever), chills, constipation or diarrhea, and a nonproductive cough (Keusch, 1991; Centers for Disease Control and Prevention, 1990). With rapid treatment, patients usually feel better within a few days.

The spectrum of illness ranges from a brief illness to an acute severe infection with central nervous system involvement and circulatory collapse. With severe infections, patient may have altered mental status, hepatitis, meningitis (Abuekteish et al., 1996), myocarditis (du Plessis et al., 1997; Hewage et al., 1994), pneumonia, arthritis (Fule and Chidgupkar, 1994), chorioamnionitis (Hedriana et al., 1995), and hemorrhage or perforation (Keusch, 1991). Untreated, up to 20 percent of patients may die from the above or other complications.[1] About 3–5 percent of patients become long-term carriers if they remain untreated. Many of these individuals never realize they were infected.

Diagnosis

A probable diagnosis can be made when a patient has a clinically compatible illness associated with a confirmed outbreak. Confirmed diagnoses require isolation of *S. typhi* from blood, stool, or another clinical specimen (Centers for Disease Control and Prevention, 1990).

Prevention

The main preventative measures for typhoid fever include avoiding potentially infectious foods and drinks and vaccination against infection. Individuals who travel to areas where typhoid is common should be vaccinated. Both oral and injectable vaccines are available (Hone et al., 1994; Klugman et al., 1996; Kollaritsch et al., 1997; Levine et al., 1996). Even those vaccinated against typhoid fever should be careful about what they eat, since the vaccine is not 100 percent effective.

Correlation with Gulf War Illnesses

Serologic markers exist to identify patients infected, either at present or in the past, with *S. typhi*. Investigation of Gulf War veterans has not detected increased antibody levels to this organism. Furthermore, in most patients this disease is either self-limited or results in severe symptoms that would precipitate immediate treatment.

Summary

Typhoid fever is caused by the bacteria *S. typhi*. This bacteria is found in most parts of the world, although it is not common in the United States, except in individuals returning from international destinations where infection is more common. Because this disease is easily diagnosed and generally lasts only a

---

[1]CDC website: http://www.cdc.gov/ncidod/diseases/bacter/typhoid.htm.

relatively short period of time, particularly with treatment, it is not a likely cause of unexplained Gulf War illnesses.

MYCOBACTERIA TUBERCULOSIS

Introduction

Mycobacterium tuberculosis is the primary bacterium responsible for causing the disease commonly known as tuberculosis (TB). The disease is present worldwide and is responsible for considerable morbidity and mortality. Tuberculosis usually exists in the form of a lung infection; however, the organism may cause disease in any organ or tissue throughout the body. The tubercule bacillus responsible for the disease is usually transmitted by the infected individual through coughing or sneezing. Although a single casual contact may transmit disease, most infections result from sustained exposures.

Epidemiologic Information

Tuberculosis has remained endemic in developing countries; however, it has reemerged as a major threat to both developing and industrialized countries over the last decade (Porter and Adams, 1994). Around the world, there are almost nine million new cases annually with more than 7,000 deaths per day attributable to TB (Rattan et al., 1998). The emergence of HIV and AIDS as a global disease has further aggravated the issue because *tuberculosis* flourishes in immunosuppressed patients (Daley, 1997; Co, 1994).

What Infected Patients Experience

Clinical signs and symptoms of tuberculosis vary considerably, ranging from a silent disease to severe systemic infection. For most individuals who contract the infection, the disease process is almost always silent, being detected only through familiar TB skin tests or x-ray findings. Occasionally, individuals with a primary TB infection may have a low-grade fever and mild anorexia. TB may remain dormant for years or even for a lifetime (Parrish et al., 1998).

Secondary tuberculosis—the phase of the disease that arises in a previously exposed individual—may also be asymptomatic although more commonly it is accompanied by insidious onset of fever, night sweats, weakness, fatigability, anorexia, and weight loss. Usually, secondary tuberculosis represents reactivation of a dormant primary infection, although exposure from exogenous sources may also occur. When the infection invades and destroys the bronchi, patients develop a productive cough, often with blood-tinged sputum and occasionally frank hemoptysis. When the disease disseminates, patients may experience differing symptoms and a fever without a clear origin.

Diagnosis

A definitive diagnosis of tuberculosis requires the identification of the tubercule bacillus. However, most individuals have been tested for *tuberculosis* using common TB skin tests (e.g., purified protein derivative, PPD) where the patient develops an infiltration (swelling) around the sight of antigen injection within 24 hours. A negative skin test, however, does not exclude the possibility of infection and patients with a past history of exposure to TB may have a positive test without an active infection. Detecting the bacillus by sputum or other culture is not always simple.

Treatment and Prevention

Preventing TB requires prompt identification and treatment of infected patients. Family members and close contacts of those found to be infected should be tested and also treated if they are shown to be positive, even if the infection is an asymptomatic primary one. A major risk factor for spread of TB is crowded living conditions and a depressed socioeconomic status.

Correlation with Gulf War Illnesses

The spectrum of disease caused by tuberculosis has been well known for centuries. The disease is recognized throughout the world, including in the Persian Gulf. It would be almost impossible to not identify some Gulf War veterans with tuberculosis given the prevalence of the disease in the population. However, the mechanism of spread, the ability to detect the infection in most individuals through simple, routinely used skin tests, and the epidemiology of the disease all suggest that tuberculosis is not the cause of undiagnosed Gulf War illnesses.

Summary

Tuberculosis is a common pulmonary infection commonly caused by repeated close contact with infected individuals. Primary infection is usually asymptomatic. However, disease reactivation occurs and the seriousness of infection is much greater in individuals with impaired immune systems (e.g., patients with HIV and those undergoing immunosuppressive treatments). Although some Gulf War veterans will undoubtedly be found to have tuberculosis, tuberculosis does not appear to be the etiology for the many individuals with undiagnosed Gulf War illnesses.

ENTERIC AGENTS: ENTEROTOXIGENIC *E. COLI, CAMPYLOBACTER, SHIGELLA,* AND OTHER *SALMONELLA*

Introduction

Infectious diarrhea continues to be a major source of international disease and death (Murray and Lopez, 1996). Although many of these infections are self-limited, some are more problematic, causing disability and even death (Frost et al., 1998). There were a number of outbreaks of diarrhea during Operation Desert Shield (Hyams et al., 1991). Such outbreaks can be particularly disabling during periods of deployment because of both the disability they inflict on the individual and the potential for spread to other individuals.

Epidemiologic Information

Hyams and colleagues collected data from U.S. troops stationed in northeastern Saudi Arabia between September and December 1990. They cultured stool from 432 individuals presenting with diarrhea, cramps, vomiting, or hematochezia. They also surveyed 2,022 soldiers in regions throughout Saudi Arabia. Researchers were able to identify a bacterial enteric pathogen in 49.5 percent of the troops with gastroenteritis. The most common bacteria were enterotoxigenic *Escherichia coli* and *Shigella sonnei.*

What Infected Patients Experience

Individuals may experience self-limited mild-to-moderate abdominal cramps with these infections, or disabling symptoms including diarrhea, cramps, vomiting, and hematochezia. Common organisms include enterotoxigenic *E. coli, Campylobacter, Shigella,* and other *Salmonella.* Each of these is slightly different.

Enterotoxigenic E. coli has an incubation period of from one to three days. Following incubation, the illness can be mild to fulminant. Most commonly patients experience mild, watery diarrhea with abdominal cramps. Vomiting is present in about half of infected individuals although it rarely is responsible for major disability. This organism is responsible for what is commonly recognized as traveler's diarrhea. The disease resolves with or without treatment; however, in the most extreme cases, fluid replacement may be necessary.

Campylobacter jejuni is second only to *Giardia* in the frequency with which it causes waterborne diarrheal diseases in the United States. After an incubation period of from two to six days, patients develop fever, cramping, abdominal pain, and diarrhea that is at first watery but later contains blood and mucus.

The diarrhea is usually mild, but not always, and lasts for a few days without therapy. Sometimes the infection can persist and patients may develop a reactive arthritis that is most commonly associated with patients carrying the HLA-B27 antigen (Altekruse, 1999).

Shigella produces an acute infectious colitis that is commonly referred to as "bacillary dysentery." The spectrum of disease is variable from mild watery diarrhea to the fatal dysentery that is more common in less-developed regions. The incubation period is from one to two days, following which some patients develop fever, some diarrhea, and some both. Patients with dysentery experience small-volume frequent stools (several per hour) consisting of blood, mucus, and pus, with abdominal cramps and tenesmus. Most patients recover over the period of up to a week, although with severe disease, they can suffer colonic perforation that can prove fatal. Very rarely patients may experience broader persistent systemic symptoms (e.g., hemolytic uremic syndrome, arthritis, seizures).

Salmonella are responsible for a number of diseases in humans. In addition to causing typhoid fever, infection can present as acute diarrhea or in more severe cases as septicemia, meningitis, reactive arthritis, osteomyelitis, and endocarditis. With respect to the gastroenteritis, the incubation period is generally from one to two days. Diarrhea (sometimes with the presence of blood) may be accompanied by nausea, vomiting, and abdominal cramps. Generally the illness is mild and self-limited, although immunosuppressed, elderly, and young patients are particularly at risk for more severe disease.

Reactive arthritis is a term used to describe joint pain and inflammation following exposure to bacterial infections, generally through either the gastrointestinal tract (most commonly following exposure to *Yersinia, Salmonella,* or *Campylobacter* species) or the genitourinary tract (most commonly associated with chlamydia infections) (Ebringer and Wilson, 2000). Many Gulf War Veterans reporting illness describe joint pain among their findings (Table 1.2).

Typical reactive arthritis patients give a history of infection within three weeks followed by arthritis in one or several joints. Some cases are accompanied by other, nonarthritic manifestations. Sometimes the diagnosis is problematic because of coexisting inflammatory processes and because in about one of four cases no infectious agent is identified (Nordstrom, 1996). Although sometimes infectious organisms may be found in the joints, laboratory findings are usually nonspecific (Beutler and Schumacher, 1997). The disease is usually self limited and resolves within six months (Nordstrom, 1996). Although some patients develop chronic arthritis, the incidence is believed to be fairly uncommon (Nordstrom, 1996; Burmester et al., 1995).

There is an extremely strong correlation between the risk of reactive arthritis and the presence of human leukocyte antigen B27 (HLA-B27) (Ebringer and Wilson, 2000; Beutler and Schumacher, 1997; al-Khonizy and Reveille, 1998; Braun and Sieper, 1996; Keat, 1999). The HLA-B27 antigen is present in approximately 8 percent of the general population (Ebringer and Wilson, 2000) with a range of 3 percent to 13 percent in the European population (Olivieri, 1998). The strength of the association between HLA-B27 can be expressed as the relative risk (of developing reactive arthritis) given the exposure (the HLA-B27 antigen). The relative risk for this association is 18, an extremely strong association.

Diagnosis

Diagnosis generally requires isolation of the organism from stool. Common laboratory techniques exist to distinguish known bacterial pathogens that infect the gastrointestinal tract.

Treatment and Prevention

Treatment depends on identifying the infecting organism and its antibiotic resistance pattern. In reality, most diseases are self-limited, particularly in healthy infected hosts. Once the bacterial resistance pattern is known, an appropriate antibiotic may be selected for those patients needing more aggressive therapy. For patients with severe diarrhea, fluid and electrolyte replacement may be indicated.

Because these are contagious, infectious diseases, prevention centers around isolation of infected individuals until the disease resolves. Furthermore, good hygiene contributes considerably to reducing the likelihood of infection.

Correlation with Gulf War Illnesses

Clearly, enteric infections occurred during the Gulf War (Hyams et al., 1991, 1995). This is not surprising given that these diseases are ubiquitous. The most common organisms identified were enterotoxigenic *E. coli* and *Shigella*. The particular strains were frequently resistant to commonly dispensed antibiotics. Although these infections occurred in the Gulf and were clearly a major problem during deployment (Hyams et al., 1991), findings were not unlike those experienced by civilians and therefore could not account for unexplained Gulf War illnesses. Some veterans likely suffer from chronic manifestations of reactive arthritis given the number of individuals who served in the Gulf and the frequency of predisposing genetic risk factors (i.e., HLA-B27). However, most patients who develop reactive arthritis achieve resolution within months.

Summary

Enteric pathogens are ubiquitous organisms known to cause diarrhea, abdominal pain, and fever. They were clearly present during service in the Persian Gulf and, in fact, accounted for a major portion of the infectious morbidity soldiers experienced during service. Most cases were mild. Except in rare cases, infections with these pathogens were self-limited. They are also easily diagnosed through common laboratory tests. Therefore, enteric pathogens could not account for the extended chronic symptoms experienced by those with unexplained Gulf War illnesses.

MENINGOCOCCUS

Introduction

Neisseria meningitidis is a gram-negative bacteria that normally populates the oropharynx (upper respiratory tract) but has the potential to cause a number of diseases, most importantly meningitis (for which it is named) and bacteremia in susceptible hosts. Healthy individuals may be carriers of the infection, and sporadic epidemiologic outbreaks continue to occur in both industrialized and developing countries.

Epidemiologic Information

Despite what has been learned about the biology and pathogenicity of *Neisseria meningitidis*, infection remains a major worldwide public health problem. The highest percentage of disease is in infants and children. In fact, *N. meningitidis* has become the leading cause of bacterial meningitis in this age group (Centers for Disease Control and Prevention, 1997a). The risk of death from disease depends on a number of factors, including the prevalence of disease, the type of infection, and the sociodemographic characteristics of the area where infection occurs (Apicella, 1995). In the United States, an 8–13 percent case-fatality rate has been reported (Centers for Disease Control and Prevention, 1997a; "Analysis of endemic meningococcal disease . . . ," 1976). In some underdeveloped countries, fatality can exceed 50 percent among septic patients (Apicella, 1995).

What Infected Patients Experience

The clinical manifestations of *N. meningitidis* infections are quite variable, ranging from a transient episode of fever to an overwhelming infection that results in death. Irrespective of the presentation, the nasopharyngeal infection that precipitates disseminated disease usually goes unrecognized or is mistaken for a mild respiratory infection. Apicella (1995) reviews the four common clinical scenarios:

- Bacteremia without sepsis—The patient has a nonspecific upper respiratory infection or rash. Although the diagnosis may be made by blood culture, the disease often resolves before the diagnosis is made.

- Meningococcemia without meningitis—The individual shows signs of sepsis (elevated white cell count, skin rashes, malaise, weakness, headache, hypotension) but without meningeal signs.

- Meningitis with or without meningococcemia—These patients have headache, fever, and accompanying meningeal signs. Cerebrospinal fluid examination suggests infection.

- Meningoencephalitic—These individuals are septic, obtunded, with meningeal signs.

With active disease, the signs a patient expresses vary widely. Petechial rashes measuring from 1–2 mm may be present, particularly on the lower half of the body. These spots may coalesce to form what appear to be ecchymoses.

Cardiovascular involvement is also well recognized with this infection, with accompanying arrhythmias, congestive heart failure, decreased tissue perfusion, and pulmonary edema. The most devastating findings are septic shock and diffuse intravascular coagulation (DIC).

Diagnosis

Because the organism commonly colonizes the oropharynx, the mere isolation of *N. meningitidis* is insufficient to confirm an infection. In fact, many healthy individuals harbor this organism. Therefore, diagnosis depends on isolation of the bacteria from what is otherwise a sterile body environment (e.g., blood, cerebrospinal fluid (CSF), pleural fluid, pericardial fluid). Bacterial culture is the standard for diagnosis, although gram-negative diplococci can be seen with abundant infections on initial Gram's stain. However, diagnosis is conventionally done by serologic measures through detection of antigens from body fluids (e.g., blood, joints, CSF). These tests (e.g., latex agglutination, counterimmunoelectrophoresis) offer accurate rapid diagnosis. These tests also enable demonstration of the specific serogroup responsible for infection. More recently, use of the polymerase chain reaction has emerged as an additional powerful diagnostic technique for meningococcal infection (Newcombe et al., 1996; Ni et al., 1992a, 1992b).

Treatment and Prevention

Particularly with the development of antibiotic resistant strains of *N. meningitidis*, efforts have been undertaken to develop vaccines using the bacterial antigens as targets for the vaccine (Oppenheim, 1997; Peltola, 1998; Saez Nieto and Vazquez, 1997; "Vaccines against meningococcal meningitis . . . ," 1994; Al-Aldeen and Cartwright, 1996). In large populations, achieving a sufficient number of protected individuals creates what is known as "herd immunity" whereby the risk of epidemics is reduced because the number of individuals harboring the infection is low, and there are no clusters of infectious individuals. In the health care setting, it is important to avoid direct contact with potentially infectious individuals, particularly those with a respiratory infection, by adhering to droplet precautions (Bolyard et al., 1998).

Secondary prevention includes chemoprophylaxis in those with known exposures. Treatment for meningococcal disease has dramatically altered the course of epidemics. Penicillin, administered either intravenously or intramuscularly, remains the first-line treatment.

Correlation with Gulf War Illnesses

Richards and colleagues (1991) confirmed four cases of *N. meningitidis* infection during Operation Desert Storm. The clinical manifestations of this disease, other than the carrier state, are generally quite dramatic, and if a significant additional population of service personnel was infected, manifestations would have been apparent and readily diagnosed. The rate of infection among those serving in the Gulf War is consistent with the rate of infection for adults in the general population. Service members were vaccinated to provide immunity, likely contributing to the low rate of infection (Lashof et al., 1996).

Summary

Neisseria meningitidis is a common bacteria that has the potential to cause serious disseminated disease in both an endemic and an epidemic fashion. Diagnostic tests exist to detect infection, and four cases were identified during the Persian Gulf occupation. Although many more individuals who served in the Persian Gulf could be found to carry the infection in the "carrier state," the mere presence of the bacteria does not imply disease. Given the dramatic clinical manifestations of disease (meningitis and sepsis), *N. meningitidis* could not account for the unexplained illnesses in Gulf War veterans.

BRUCELLA

Introduction

Brucellosis, also known as undulant fever, is a systemic bacterial infection that in humans results from contact with infected animals or ingestion of infected animal products, including milk.[2] The disease was first recognized over a century ago during the Crimean War as causing "Mediterranean gastric remittent fever." Four recognized species result in human disease, including *B. melitensis* (the usual animal hosts are sheep and goats), *B. abortus* (the usual animal hosts are cattle), *B. canis* (the usual animal hosts are dogs), and *B. suis* (the usual animal hosts are swine). The bacteria is a small, nonmotile, nonencapsulated, gram-negative coccobacillus. Brucellosis is an enteric fever that produces primarily systemic complaints often with associated gastrointestinal manifestations. Because of the way the bacterium is spread and its worldwide distribution, it has been responsible for considerable morbidity among humans and animals.

Epidemiologic Information

Brucellosis continues to be a major source of disease among humans and domestic animals. Incidence and prevalence vary from country to country, although bovine brucellosis, caused mainly by *B. abortus*, is still the most widespread infection. In humans, ovine/caprine brucellosis caused by *B. melitensis* is the most important clinically apparent disease, particularly in the Mediterranean, western Asia, and parts of Africa and Latin America (Corbell, 1997). For example, in the southern region of Saudi Arabia, a recent study found that 19 percent of the population had serologic evidence of exposure to Brucella antigen, and 2.3 percent of individuals had active disease (Alballa, 1995).

The reported incidence of brucellosis varies from less than 0.01 per 100,000 to over 200 per 100,000 population (Corbell, 1997). Incidence of infection is high in some areas, such as Kuwait and Saudi Arabia. Areas where rates appear low may reflect underreporting rather than actual low incidence of disease. Differences in various countries may also reflect food preparation customs, public health measures, including pasteurization of dairy products, and the extent of contact with potentially infected animals.

---

[2]CDC website: http://www.cdc.gov/od/oc/media/brucello.htm.

What Infected Patients Experience

Symptom onset, generally starting about two to eight weeks following exposure, can be either acute or insidious, with equal likelihood. Patient symptoms are generally nonspecific and include fever, sweats, malaise, anorexia, headache, and back pain. These nonspecific findings can be misinterpreted as being a benign viral illness. Without treatment, patients experience an undulating febrile pattern, hence its common name "undulant fever." Patients may have other complaints including depression and an unusual taste in the mouth. Reports of physical findings vary and are more elusive with about 10 percent experiencing lymphadenopathy, 20–30 percent having splenomegaly, and 10–60 percent with hepatomegaly (Young, 1995a, 1995b; Kaye, 1991).

Gastrointestinal symptoms are usually present but may or may not be severe even though brucellosis is an enteric infection. Usually the generalized findings predominate. Up to 60 percent of patients report joint problems (Young, 1995a), particularly the hips, knees, and ankles. Bone scans may show inflammation, although definitive radiological evidence of damage is a late finding. Neurologic manifestations of the disease include meningitis, encephalitis, peripheral neuropathy, and psychosis. Central nervous system involvement is less common. A small fraction (2 percent) of patients experience endocarditis although this is the most worrisome manifestation and can be fatal because of valvular destruction, if not recognized soon enough. Myocarditis and pericarditis can also occur. About a quarter of patients have some respiratory symptoms ranging from those commonly associated with nonspecific viral illness to bronchopneumonia, lung abscesses, and pleural effusions. Genitourinary findings are unusual but can occur.

A chronic form of brucellosis is recognized when a patient has ill health for a period of at least 12 months. These individuals have relapsing illness and most have persisting focal infection, such as in bone, spleen or liver (Young, 1995a).

Diagnosis

Because the clinical presentation is not specific, laboratory confirmation must be made to arrive at a definitive diagnosis. Routine laboratory tests (e.g., white cell count) generally do not suggest the presence of a bacterial infection. For patients with acute disease, blood (or tissue) culture remains the diagnostic standard (Corbell, 1997; Gad El-Rab and Kambal, 1998; Gaviria-Ruiz and Cardona-Castro, 1995). Because the presence of *Brucella* cannot be demonstrated through standard culture techniques, serologic tests can be used to establish a presumptive diagnosis (Gad El-Rab and Kambal, 1998; Barbuddhe et al., 1994; Barbuddhe and Yadava, 1997; Young, 1991).

Prevention

The key to elimination of brucellosis in humans is the eradication, or at least the control, of the disease in animals. The greater risk is the consumption of infected animal products, rather than the handling of animals (Cooper, 1992). Individuals working in higher risk venues, such as farmers, veterinarians, and other animal health professionals, should receive specific education on hygienic precautions to avoid infection and training to recognize the possibility that findings might be secondary to *Brucella*. A safe and effective human vaccine is not available at present and those that have been developed have been fraught with problems (Corbell, 1997).

Correlation with Gulf War Illnesses

Brucellosis is a bacterial infection with a worldwide distribution. Infection occurs by consuming or handling infected animals or animal products such as dairy products. The CDC reports a fairly high incidence of brucellosis in areas involved with Operation Desert Storm and Operation Desert Shield. However, brucellosis is a bacterial disease with a known cause that can be diagnosed by currently available techniques. Clearly, many of the nonspecific findings associated with brucellosis have similarities with undiagnosed Gulf War illnesses; however, because diagnostic tests exist for brucellosis and veterans have not shown evidence of infection, brucellosis is not likely to explain the undiagnosed illnesses in Gulf War veterans. Given the natural prevalence of brucellosis, some individuals may actually have a chronic infection unrelated to their service in the Gulf.

Summary

Brucellosis is a zoonotic bacterial disease that infects humans through contact with infected animals and animal products, particularly dairy products. The bacteria have a worldwide distribution, and some species are prominent in the Middle East. Patients may either present with an acute infection or experience a more insidious course. Infection usually manifests with a number of nondiagnostic findings, including GI, orthopedic, neurologic, cardiovascular, and pulmonary symptoms. Many of these findings have some similarity to reported symptoms in patients with undiagnosed Gulf War illnesses. However, brucellosis is diagnosable through culture, serologic (presumptive), and molecular methods. Investigation of ill individuals following Gulf War service has not revealed evidence of infection with this bacterium.

CHOLERA

Introduction

Vibrio cholerae is a gram-negative comma-shaped bacterium that has been known for many years to cause diarrheal illness secondary to intestinal infection. The infection is frequently mild or asymptomatic, but it can be severe. Approximately 5 percent of infected persons have severe disease (cholera) characterized by profuse watery diarrhea, vomiting, and leg cramps. In these individuals, rapid loss of body fluids leads to dehydration and shock; without aggressive treatment, death can occur within hours.

Epidemiologic Information

In the United States, cholera was common during in the 1800s. The disease has been virtually eliminated by modern sewage and water treatment systems. However, travelers to areas with epidemic cholera may be exposed to the cholera bacterium.

During epidemics, many individuals excrete large volumes of stool containing abundant vibrio organisms. This excrement can contaminate the water supply that is used for washing, drinking, cooking, and swimming.

What Infected Patients Experience

The pathogenicity of cholera results from an enterotoxin that the bacteria produces. The organism itself does not result in patient illness. The enterotoxin activates enzymes in the small bowel that result in massive secretion of fluid into the bowel, overwhelming the normal reabsorptive capacity of the colon. Patients produce large volumes of dilute, relatively clear diarrhea. Untreated, patients experience signs of dehydration with dry mouth, recessed eyes, a thready pulse, lethargy, and anuria. With adequate therapy in the form of fluid replacement, almost all patients survive. With inadequate treatment, death rates may approach 50 percent, mostly from dehydration and its consequences.

Diagnosis

When cholera is suspected, definitive diagnosis can be made through microbiologic examination of the stool. The organism can be identified by trained microbiologists on examination of fresh stool, and the bacterium can be cultured using readily available media. Newer immunologic and molecular mechanisms now exist to aid in the diagnosis of this disease (Hoshino et al., 1998; Varela et al., 1994; Hasan et al., 1994; Qadri et al., 1994).

Treatment and Prevention

A short-acting vaccine is available for individuals exposed to cholera; however, the vaccine is not usually recommended for individuals traveling to areas (e.g., Latin America) where cholera is commonly found.

Treatment for cholera is supportive, with replacement of fluids and electrolytes through intravenous and oral therapy. When recognized and treated, patients recover from their infection without long-term consequences.

Correlation with Gulf War Illnesses

Cholera produces an acute, devastating diarrheal illness that would be hard to miss. The findings (or lack thereof) in patients with undiagnosed Gulf War illnesses are not consistent with cholera.

Summary

Cholera is an acute diarrheal illness that places the patient at serious threat of mortality from dehydration if the fluids lost are not properly replaced. However, with timely treatment, patients recover from the infection without long-term sequelae. Given the acute nature of the disease, cholera is not consistent with undiagnosed Gulf War illnesses.

Chapter Five

VIRAL DISEASES

VIRAL HEPATITIS

Introduction

Hepatitis literally means inflammation of the liver. This section focuses on viral hepatitis, infection caused by a group of viruses that primarily affect the liver. Important forms of hepatitis to be discussed include hepatitis A (HAV), hepatitis B (HBV), hepatitis C (HCV). Discussions address each of these infections because although they all cause "hepatitis," their clinical pictures differ considerably.

Although other hepatitis viruses are gaining more prominence and are present in the Middle East, they are not discussed in detail here. The only one of these viruses that poses a potential threat is hepatitis E, a virus that clinically looks like HAV, causes an acute infection, and is spread by the fecal-oral route (Oldfield et al., 1991; Burans et al., 1994).

Epidemiologic Information

Hepatitis A is usually transmitted by the fecal-oral route. Infectious outbreaks occur where there is exposure to infected water or food (e.g., shellfish, commercial food preparation where an employee does not follow standard food handling guidelines) (Bean et al., 1996). Only in rare circumstances is this infection transmitted through parenteral routes. The Centers for Disease Control and Prevention estimates that between 125,000 and 200,000 infections occur annually in the United States, of which about 70 percent of adults are symptomatic. In rare circumstances (about 100 cases/year), HAV causes a lethal fulminant hepatitis. Serologic testing reveals that about one-third of Americans have evidence of past exposure to the virus. Periodic outbreaks occur. Groups at particularly high risk include household and sexual contacts of infected individuals, those who travel internationally, particularly to destinations where the infection is endemic, American Indians, and people in close contact with infected patients, particularly during an outbreak. HAV is endemic in the Middle East, Africa, Asia, and Central and South America where the serologic prevalence of exposure to HAV has been reported to be as high as 96 percent (Oldfield et al., 1991; Heintges and Wand, 1997; el-Hazmi, 1989a).

Hepatitis B virus transmission occurs via parenteral routes with transmission through contact with infected blood, through sexual transmission, and from mother to child in the perinatal period. Risk groups include those who use intravenous drugs, individuals sexually active with multiple partners, homosexual men, infants born to infected mothers, hemodialysis patients, and healthcare workers. Hepatitis B is more common among lower socioeconomic groups; however, it is observed among all economic strata. The CDC estimates that there are between 140,000 and 320,000 infections annually in the United States with about half of them being symptomatic. Serologic evidence indicates a prevalence of between 1 and 1.25 million individuals with chronic Hepatitis B virus infection.

Hepatitis B is also common in areas where troops were deployed during Operation Desert Storm (Hyams et al., 1989; McCarthy et al., 1989). Serologic evidence suggests that the prevalence of Hepatitis B infection in Saudi Arabia is about 17 percent (Oldfield et al., 1991; el-Hazmi, 1989b). The incidence of HBV infection has decreased over the last decade as a result of the availability of vaccines and reduced high-risk behaviors.

Hepatitis C has been only recently recognized as a specific entity (Alter et al., 1998). The virus is responsible for the majority of cases of what was previously called non-A, non-B viral hepatitis. The CDC estimates that between 35,000 to 180,000 infections occur annually in the United States, of which up to 30 percent are symptomatic. Routes of transmission are similar to those for hepatitis B although risk factors differ. An estimated four million Americans are infected with HCV (Alter, 1997). This virus is also endemic in the Middle East (Al-Arabi et al., 1987; Bassily et al., 1983). Although the blood supply was previously responsible for a large number of transfusion-associated infections, the availability of commercially available screening tests has dramatically reduced this risk and improved the overall safety of the supply.

What Infected Patients Experience

The main clinical features of the three types of viral hepatitis are similar with the most common features being fatigue, abdominal discomfort, jaundice (yellowing of the skin and whites of the eyes), and loss of appetite.

Hepatitis A does not develop a chronic state although about 15 percent of patients experience a prolonged or relapsing course. Patients may have intermittent diarrhea and nausea. IgM anti-HAV antibody (indicating acute infection) appears approximately four weeks after exposure and rarely persists longer than six months.

Hepatitis B infections present with similar symptoms usually several weeks following infection. The findings are initially similar to those described for HAV, including a rare patient with fulminant disease who may die acutely from the infection. However, there are between 8,000 and 32,000 new chronic infections per year resulting in between 5,000 and 6,000 deaths annually from liver failure and liver cancer. Patients with chronic hepatitis are at risk for primary liver cancer (hepatocellular carcinoma) (Hoofnagle and di Bisceglie, 1997).

Hepatitis C has a similar presentation to the other viruses; however, the risk of chronic infection is much higher with this virus (at least 85 to 90 percent). Consequently, chronic liver disease develops in the majority of patients and the risk of death from chronic liver disease is much higher in these patients (about 8,000 to 10,000 deaths per year) (Hoofnagle, 1997).

Diagnosis

Diagnosis of the common hepatitis infections is easily made through laboratory tests. In fact, the availability of these techniques has dramatically reduced the risk of transfusion-transmitted disease because these tests are commonly used to screen all blood donors. There are tests that will diagnose current, chronic, and past hepatitis infections, depending on the patient's condition and the virus involved.

Treatment and Prevention

Treatment for HAV is primarily supportive because of its self-limited nature (Koff, 1998; Lemon, 1997). Treating HBV and HCV infections is also supportive; however, because of the risk of chronic liver disease, including hepatocellular carcinoma and cirrhosis, interferon and other medications are available to retard the development of the long-term complications of chronic disease. For patients who develop end-stage liver disease, surgical interventions can reduce the morbidity of disease. Liver transplant remains an option for those patients who are refractory to other treatments and who develop life-threatening liver failure. Newer treatments and complementary therapies continue to be developed (Bonkovsky, 1997; Brady 1997; Damen et al., 1998; Everhart et al., 1997; Inchauspe, 1997).

Prevention of those hepatitis infections transmitted by the fecal-oral route involves standard hygiene and sanitation techniques. It is important for food handlers to adhere to proper food preparation standards. Immunoglobulin can be given to individuals prophylactically or patients with known recent exposure can receive anti-HA immunoglobulin. Recently, a hepatitis A vaccine became available that reduces the risk of HAV disease. Immune globulin is also available to the nonimmune patient who is exposed. Vaccines for HBV have been available since 1982 and have been instrumental in reducing the risk of infection from this virus (Zannolli and Morgese, 1997; Zimmerman et al., 1997). Infants and children are now routinely vaccinated, and recommendations exist to vaccinate others in high-risk groups (e.g., healthcare workers, homosexual men). Blood and tissue donor screening also reduces the risk of transmission to recipients. Community programs can reduce transmission through recreational intravenous drugs. For HCV, screening of blood and tissue donors and reduction of risky behaviors can help reduce the transmission rate. A vaccination to prevent transmission of HCV is not yet available.

Correlation with Gulf War Illnesses

Although all the forms of hepatitis discussed in this review exist in the Middle East, the primary concern during the deployment centered on those infections that are transmitted via the fecal-oral route. Particularly because the risk of transmission is increased when individuals live in close proximity, this was a concern during Operation Desert Storm. However, because many patients infected with the hepatitis viruses are symptomatic, the absence of specific symptoms (e.g., jaundice) and the absence of an increased prevalence of laboratory tests positive for infection suggest that hepatitis is not responsible for the symptoms experienced by individuals with undiagnosed Gulf War illnesses. Immune gamma-globulin was used in service members to prevent hepatitis A infection (Lashof et al., 1996). However, given the high prevalence of these diseases, it is not surprising that some veterans, like civilians, will be infected with hepatitis viruses through other routes of exposure.

Summary

The group of hepatitis viruses primarily infect the liver with resultant gastrointestinal and systemic manifestations. These infections are common in the Middle East and in the United States. Although it is expected that some veterans will have hepatitis, the presence of the infection does not imply that military service is the etiology of the exposure.

CRIMEAN-CONGO HEMORRHAGIC FEVER

Introduction

Crimean-Congo hemorrhagic fever is caused by a virus that is part of the Bunyaviridae family, genus Nairovirus. This infection is emerging as an important zoonotic disease (animal disease transmitted to humans). The virus has been identified throughout sub-Saharan Africa, the Middle East, Asia, and Eastern Europe.

The disease is transmitted from the bite of the *Hyalomma* tick, although nosocomial and household transmission to humans has been observed. Cattle, sheep, and wild hares appear to be the most important animal reservoirs for the virus although *Hyalomma* are attracted to humans.

Epidemiologic Information

The virus has been identified in outbreaks in the Soviet Union, Bulgaria, Pakistan, Iraq, Dubai, Kuwait, and the United Arab Emirates (Gubler and Clark, 1995; Kwiatkowski and Marsh, 1997; Kitua, 1997; Soares and Rodrigues, 1998; Connor et al., 1998; Greenwood, 1997; Facer and Tanner, 1997; Dubois and Pereira da Silva, 1995). The disease is fairly common among some populations in Iraq. Tikriti and colleagues observed that nearly 30 percent of animal breeders tested had antibodies to the virus (Tikriti et al., 1981).

Although a less common route of infection, as indicated, nosocomial infection has been observed in most of the geographic areas in which the virus is endemic. When infection has occurred, there have been high fatality rates. This means that strict blood and body fluid precautions must be taken when infection is even suspected.

What Infected Patients Experience

The incubation period for the virus ranges from three to 12 days, followed by sudden onset of severe headaches. Fever, accompanied by shaking chills, is also present initially or shortly thereafter. The fever usually lasts for about a week or slightly longer with about half of those affected experiencing a 12- to 48-hour afebrile period sometime in the middle of the illness (i.e., a double peaked fever curve) (Oldfield et al., 1991).

The fever is frequently accompanied by muscle aches (particularly in the low back and legs), sore throat, and photophobia. Many patients have accompanying nausea and vomiting. Gastrointestinal complaints, in half of infected patients, include diffuse abdominal pain and diarrhea. Patients may also develop hepatomegaly (enlarged liver) and right upper quadrant abdominal pain. Facial flushing, possibly involving the upper torso, also occurs. Bradycardia is also observed.

After several days, a petechial rash develops that is associated with epistaxis, hematemesis, and melena (Oldfield et al., 1991), which are manifestations of the ensuing disseminated intravascular coagulation (DIC). The fatality rate for this virus is between 13 and 70 percent, occurring between days six and 14 of the illness (Oldfield et al., 1991; Schwarz et al., 1997).

Diagnosis

Laboratory tests and serologic assays are available that specifically identify the virus and detect host response to the virus (Burt et al., 1994). More recently, a polymerase chain reaction molecular diagnostic protocol has emerged (Burt et al., 1998).

Treatment and Prevention

The treatment for infected patients is primarily supportive. However, recent efforts have shown promising results for specific therapies, including ribavirin and specific intravenous immunoglobulin (Centers for Disease Control and Prevention, 1995; Fisher-Hoch et al., 1995; Tignor and Hanham, 1993; Vassilenko et al., 1990).

Prevention involves reducing exposure to the ticks in endemic areas through the use of pesticides (e.g., DEET) and protective clothing. Individuals should look for and remove ticks on their bodies. In the clinical setting, including the clinical laboratory, methods must be taken to avoid contact with blood and body fluids of potentially infected patients.

Correlation with Gulf War Illnesses

There were no identified cases of Crimean-Congo hemorrhagic fever among individuals who served in the Gulf War (Richards et al., 1991). Because this disease is profoundly symptomatic in infected individuals and diagnostic tests are available to identify infection, Crimean-Congo hemorrhagic fever is unlikely to be the cause of the chronic illnesses experienced by some Gulf War veterans.

Summary

Crimean-Congo hemorrhagic fever is a viral infection that is well known in the areas where U.S. troops served in the Gulf War. The infection is passed to humans from the bite of the *Hyalomma* tick, but nosocomial and household transmission have also been observed. No individuals studied show evidence of contracting Crimean-Congo hemorrhagic fever and the clinical presentation is inconsistent with what is observed in patients with undiagnosed Gulf War illnesses.

WEST NILE FEVER

Introduction

West Nile fever is caused by a virus that is part of the Flaviviridae family. There are nearly 70 different viruses in this group, formerly termed group B arboviruses, of which nearly half are known to cause illness in humans. The World Health Organization defines arboviruses (arthropod-borne viruses) as a group as those "which are maintained in nature principally, or to an important extent, through biological transmission between susceptible vertebrate hosts by hematophagous arthropods; they multiply and produce viremia in the vertebrates, multiply in the tissues of arthropods, and are passed on to new vertebrates by the bites of arthropods after a period of extrinsic incubation" (Sanford, 1991). Common viruses in this classification, in addition to West Nile, include yellow fever, dengue, Japanese encephalitis, St. Louis encephalitis, and tick-borne encephalitis viruses. These viruses are generally spread by mosquitoes or ticks; human-to-human spread does not occur. Infection with these viruses does not produce a unique clinical picture. Therefore, travel to an endemic area and laboratory tests are important for identifying a specific infection.

West Nile virus is a mosquito-borne virus found most commonly in Africa, France, India, Indonesia, the Middle East, and Soviet countries. In 1999, a West-Nile-like virus was identified in patients living in the Northeast United States. The bird is the primary host and the principal vector is *Culex univittatus*. However, other mosquitoes are known to carry the virus, including *Culex pipiens*, *Culex antennatus*, and *Culex tritaeniorhynchus* (Asia). Other animal reservoirs are not part of the virus's normal life cycle.

Epidemiologic Information

West Nile fever is common in the Middle East with most individuals exposed as children. Children experience a nondescript viral illness with fever that is rarely diagnosed. Neighboring Israel also experiences infection although there, it is more likely the young adult than the child who becomes infected. Spread occurs primarily in the summer months when the mosquito population increases.

What Infected Patients Experience

The incubation period for the virus is between one and six days. After the incubation period, the patient's temperature rises rapidly to between 101°F and 104°F accompanied with nonspecific symptoms associated with fever, including drowsiness, a severe frontal headache, ocular pain, and abdominal and back pain. In addition, patients experience facial flushing, conjunctival injection (red eyes), and coating of the tongue, accompanied by moderate lymph node enlargement (occipital, axillary, inguinal) with some tenderness (Sanford, 1991). About one third of patients experience chills. Half of infected patients experience a rash between one and four days after onset of the illness that lasts from a few hours to until the fever breaks. In most patients, the illness is self-limited, resolving over a few days with lymph node enlargement decreasing over a few months. Rarely are long-term complications observed, and fatalities are extremely rare.

Diagnosis

Nonspecific laboratory tests include leukopenia (total white blood cell count less than 4000/µL). Definitive diagnostic tests exist, in the form of viral isolation (during infection) or the identification of a rising specific antibody titer.

Treatment and Prevention

For infected patients, the goal is to treat the symptoms. There are no specific treatments for West Nile fever. Prevention involves reducing exposure to the mosquito population in endemic areas.

Correlation with Gulf War Illnesses

There was one confirmed case of West Nile fever among individuals serving in the Gulf War (Hyams et al., 1995; Richards et al., 1991). Furthermore, the insect vector was identified in the area (Cope et al., 1996). However, the use of insecticides and troop deployment in the cooler months led to conditions that were not favorable to the transmission of this virus. Because this disease is self-limited and diagnostic tests are available to identify infection, West Nile fever is unlikely to be the cause of the chronic illnesses experienced by some Gulf War veterans.

Summary

West Nile fever is a viral infection common in Africa, the Middle East, some areas within Europe, India, Indonesia, and in Soviet countries. It is normally passed from mosquito to bird and back to mosquito. Human involvement in this cycle is incidental. West Nile fever is a self-limited febrile illness; few patients experience any long-term sequelae from the infection. Infection is easily diagnosed through common laboratory tests. Although one individual serving in the Gulf War did contract West Nile fever, the clinical presentation is inconsistent with what is observed in patients with undiagnosed Gulf War illnesses.

SINDBIS

Introduction

Sindbis is a vector-borne alphavirus that produces a disease characterized by fever, rash, and polyarthritis. This virus, native to Africa, Scandinavia, former Soviet countries, Australia, and Asia (Norder et al., 1996), is part of the Togaviridae family, which includes the more commonly recognized eastern equine encephalitis and western equine encephalitis viruses. The most recognized member of the Togaviridae family is the virus that causes rubella. The virus is a positive-stranded RNA virus.

Epidemiologic Information

Sindbis was first described in 1961, during an outbreak of five cases in Uganda (Niklasson, 1998). The Sindbis virus exists among birds, transmitted primarily by *Culex* mosquitoes. A South African study demonstrated the clear association between human disease outbreaks and excessive rainfall, particularly when water stands in usually dry areas. Infection rates may approach 15 percent of the susceptible population in particularly favorable settings. Sindbis shares its vector with that of the West Nile virus. The pattern of this vector is discussed in greater detail in the West Nile virus section above. Because of this common viral vector, in the Middle East it is common to find individuals who are positive for exposure to Sindbis to also be positive for exposure to West Nile virus.

What Infected Patients Experience

Sindbis usually presents as a sudden onset of low-grade fever after an incubation period of usually less than one week (Niklasson, 1998). Patients experience accompanying myalgias, malaise, and arthralgia that affect the joints and tendons. The joints involved include the wrist (50 percent), fingers (18 percent), hips (26 percent), knee (42 percent), and ankle (62 percent). Swollen joints do not show significant fluid accumulation. The key feature of Sindbis is the maculopapular nonpruritic (6 percent of patients report itchiness) rash on the trunk and extremities that becomes vesicular, particularly on the extremities. The papules are approximately 3 mm in diameter. The rash is present for an average of one week (range 1 to 21 days). Although the rash and fever are almost always gone after three weeks, arthralgia may persist for many months in some cases (Niklasson, 1988). Fatal cases of Sindbis have not been reported.

Diagnosis

The virus can be isolated from blood or vesicle fluid during the acute phase of the infection. Nonspecific laboratory tests include mild leukopenia and elevation of acute phase reactants. In addition to these nonspecific findings, definitive diagnostic tests exist, particularly the identification of a rising specific antibody titer.

Treatment and Prevention

As with other members of this virus group, treatment is supportive and with time (usually a short period but perhaps up to several months), the symptoms resolve. Prevention, as with other arboviruses, centers on decreased exposure to the potentially infective mosquito through the use of repellants and the wearing of clothing that covers the body, particularly when the mosquito population is abundant (Peters and Dalrymple, 1990).

Correlation with Gulf War Illnesses

There were no identified cases of Sindbis among individuals who served in the Gulf War (Richards et al., 1991). The presentation and course of this disease is not consistent with the findings of those individuals with undiagnosed illnesses associated with Gulf War service, even though some of the initial findings may bear a similarity to Gulf War veterans' symptoms. Sindbis, therefore, is unlikely to be the cause of the chronic illnesses experienced by Gulf War veterans.

Summary

Sindbis is an arbovirus that produces fever, rash, and polyarthritis. The virus is transmitted to humans through *Culex* mosquitoes. No cases of sindbis have been identified among individuals serving in the Gulf War and the chronic symptoms among Gulf War veterans with undiagnosed illnesses are not generally characteristic of this infection.

RIFT VALLEY FEVER

Introduction

Rift Valley fever is an acute, fever-causing viral disease that affects domestic animals (e.g., cattle, buffalo, sheep, goats, and camels) and humans. Rift Valley fever is most commonly associated with mosquito-borne epidemics during years of heavy rainfall.[1] Rift Valley fever virus is a Phlebovirus in the family Bunyaviridae. Other viruses within this family include California encephalitis virus, Crimean-Congo hemorrhagic fever, and hantavirus.

People get Rift Valley fever from the bites of mosquitoes (*Aedes mcintoshi, Culex pipiens, Eretmapodites chrysogaster, Aedes caballus, Aedes circumluteolus, Culex theileri*) and possibly other blood-sucking insects that serve as vectors. People can also get the disease if they are exposed to either the blood or other body fluids of infected animals. Therefore, increased risk of infection is seen in farmers, veterinarians, and others who handle infected animals and carcasses. Individuals handling laboratory specimens have also become infected, suggesting an aerosol transmission route.

Epidemiologic Information

Rift Valley fever occurs in regions of eastern and southern Africa where sheep and cattle are raised, although the infection is also seen in most countries of sub-Saharan Africa and Madagascar. The virus primarily affects livestock and can cause disease in a large number of domestic animals. The presence of a Rift Valley fever epizootic can lead to an epidemic in people exposed to diseased animals.

Infection is transmitted from generation to generation of mosquitoes through the eggs of infected mosquitoes. It is possible for infected eggs to remain dormant in soil for extended periods of time, only to emerge when moisture returns, as in the case of heavy rains or man-made events that alter environmental moisture.

What Infected Patients Experience

Most patients experience a nonspecific febrile reaction. After an incubation period of three to six days, the patient's temperature rises rapidly to 101°F to 104°F. Initial onset of fever may be accompanied by chills, malaise, headache, retroorbital pain, and backache. Some patients may experience nausea and

---

[1]CDC website: http://www.cdc.gov/ncidod/dvrd/rvf/rvf.htm.

vomiting (Arthur et al., 1993). Later, patients may experience anorexia, epigastric pain, and photophobia. Patients may experience defervescence after two to three days, followed by a second temperature spike before resolution. For most patients, Rift Valley fever is considered a benign, self-limited disease.

Between 1 and 5 percent of individuals develop ocular problems, including retinitis and vasculitis that results in some degree of permanent visual loss among about half the affected patients. Rarely (in about 1 percent), at the end of the febrile period, patients develop severe fulminant disease that can include encephalitis, hemorrhage, jaundice, and hepatitis. When such serious manifestations occur, 50 percent or more may die.

Diagnosis

Rift Valley fever can be diagnosed easily through laboratory testing. During the infectious period, the virus can be isolated from blood (in about 75 percent of patients) and by detection of antibodies that are present four to 14 days after onset of disease, coinciding with clinical improvement.

Treatment and Prevention

Treatment of patients is symptomatic; there are no specific treatments for Rift Valley fever. Prevention involves avoidance of mosquitoes when traveling to endemic areas and reducing exposure to potentially infected animal products and laboratory specimens.

Correlation with Gulf War Illnesses

There were no identified cases of Rift Valley fever among individuals who served in the Gulf War (Richards et al., 1991). The insect vector was identified in the area (Cope et al., 1996). However, the use of insecticides and troop deployment in the cooler months led to conditions that were not favorable to the transmission of this virus. Because this disease is self-limited and diagnostic tests are available to identify infection, Rift Valley fever is unlikely to be the cause of the chronic illnesses experienced by some Gulf War veterans.

Summary

Rift Valley fever is a viral infection common in areas in and around the Persian Gulf and Africa. There was concern that U.S. service members may have been exposed. The virus is normally passed from mosquito to animals, particularly sheep and cattle, and back to mosquito. Human infection occurs through mosquito bites, from handling infected animal tissues, and from failure to take adequate precautions when handling infectious laboratory specimens. Rift Valley fever is generally a self-limited febrile illness, although a small percentage of individuals experience a fulminant infection with high mortality. Infection is easily diagnosed through common laboratory tests. No individuals studied show evidence of contracting Rift Valley fever (Hyams et al., 1995) and the clinical presentation is inconsistent with what is observed in patients with undiagnosed Gulf War illnesses.

RABIES

Introduction

Rabies is caused by a number of different viruses within the Rhabdoviridae family and was first recognized more than 4,000 years ago. Although the virus has been classically associated with dogs and dog bites, rabies can affect a large number of wild and domesticated animal species. Because the virus exists in the Gulf region, some individuals raised the question whether rabies might contribute to the illness experienced among Gulf War veterans.

Epidemiologic Information

Rabies has been reported on all continents except Australia and Antarctica. Over the last half century, there has been a dramatic decrease in rabies among domestic animals in the United States. This has been accompanied by the consequent decrease in human cases to fewer than two cases per year in the 1960s and 1970s and fewer than one case per year during the 1980s (Reid-Sanden et al., 1990). Therefore, the likelihood of exposure to a rabid domestic animal is very low, although many possible exposures occur that constitute the basis for antirabies treatment (Helmick, 1983).

Only about 1,000 rabies deaths are reported to the World Health Organization annually, even though the annual incidence of rabies is believed to be about 30,000 cases. The disease is most common in Southeast Asia, the Philippines, Africa, the Indian subcontinent, and tropical areas of South America (Corey, 1991).

Rabies among wild animals (especially skunks, raccoons, and bats) has accounted for more than 85 percent of all reported cases of animal rabies every year since 1976 in the United States (Gonzalez-Ruiz et al., 1994). Wild animals are now the most important potential source of infection for both humans and domestic animals in the United States. However, in much of the rest of the world, including most of Asia, Africa, and Latin America, the dog remains the major species with rabies and the major source of rabies among humans (Centers for Disease Control and Prevention, 1991).

Rabies is transmitted to humans only when the virus is introduced through open cuts or wounds in skin or mucous membranes via bites or infected animal saliva. The likelihood of contracting rabies varies with the type of exposures.

What Infected Patients Experience

After the incubation period of weeks to many months, the disease initially presents with a nonspecific prodromal phase in from 50 to 80 percent of patients. This period lasts from one to 10 days. Patients experience severe fever, headache, malaise, myalgias, easy fatigability, and cough. Early neurologic involvement may precipitate apprehension, anxiety, agitation, irritability, nervousness, insomnia, psychiatric abnormalities, or depression (Fishbein and Bernard, 1995).

Following the conclusion of the prodromal phase, the patient progresses to the encephalitic or acute neurologic phase. At this stage, which lasts usually from two to seven days, neurologic manifestations are extreme. Almost all patients die from one or more systemic complication of rabies.

Diagnosis

At first, the laboratory findings are generally either normal or nonspecific. The specific diagnosis requires either isolation of the virus from infected body fluids or the demonstration of serologic evidence for infection. Clinically, it is difficult to distinguish rabies from other viral infections that produce similar findings (Corey, 1991; Fishbein and Bernard, 1995).

Treatment and Prevention

Because rabies is virtually 100 percent fatal without intervention, prevention is critical. The most important means of prevention is the control of the virus in animal populations, particularly domestic animals. Pre- and postexposure prophylaxis is also important in preventing the devastating consequences of this disease.

Correlation with Gulf War Illnesses

The clinical findings, as discussed above, are not consistent with the findings of individuals who have undiagnosed Gulf War illnesses. Although some of the early signs and symptoms of rabies may have some resemblance to Gulf War illnesses, the 100 percent case-fatality rate is entirely inconsistent with chronic symptoms.

Summary

Rabies is a serious infection, transmitted to humans through the bite of infected animals. This infection has a very high case-fatality rate. Although endemic in most parts of the world, including areas where U.S. military visited during the Gulf War, rabies cannot be the etiology for unexplained Gulf War illnesses. There are good diagnostic tests for rabies. That, combined with the clinical outcome of the disease, excludes this infection from the list of possible causes for unexplained symptoms in Gulf War veterans.

DENGUE

Introduction

Dengue fever is caused by a virus that is part of the Flaviviridae family. There are nearly 70 different viruses in this group, formerly termed group B arboviruses, of which nearly half are known to cause illness in humans. Other common viruses in this classification include yellow fever, West Nile, Japanese encephalitis, St. Louis encephalitis, and tick-borne encephalitis viruses. The most common infection in humans is caused by the dengue virus, of which there are four types. Flaviviruses are generally spread by mosquitoes or ticks; human-to-human spread does not occur. Infection with these viruses does not produce a unique clinical picture. Therefore, travel to an endemic area and laboratory tests are important for identifying specific infection.

Dengue and dengue hemorrhagic fever (DHF) are caused by infection with one of four antigenically distinct, virus serotypes (DEN-1, DEN-2, DEN-3, and DEN-4). Once infected with one of these serotypes, the individual develops specific immunity. However, cross-immunity does not develop. It is theoretically possible, therefore, for an individual to be infected four times, each time with a different serotype.

Dengue is mostly seen in tropical urban areas. As with other members of the Flaviviridae family, the virus is transmitted through mosquito bites, specifically *Aedes aegypti*. This mosquito, a domestic, day-biting mosquito, prefers to feed on humans (Gubler and Clark, 1995). In some parts of the world (mostly Asia and Oceania) other vectors have been implicated: *A. albopictus, A. scutellaris, and A. polynesiensis.*

Epidemiologic Information

Dengue is the most important mosquito-borne viral disease, affecting humans with a distribution comparable to that of malaria. Approximately 2.5 billion people are living in areas at risk for epidemic transmission (Gubler and Clark, 1995). Tens of millions of cases of dengue fever occur annually along with up to hundreds of thousands of cases of dengue hemorrhagic fever.

What Infected Patients Experience

Dengue infection can produce a broad range of clinical findings. Common findings, described during an outbreak in U.S. troops during Operation Restore Hope in Somalia during 1992–1993 include fever (mean temperature on admission in this group was 102°F) (100 percent), chills (93 percent), myalgias (84 percent), headache (86 percent), retro-orbital pain (53 percent), rash (49 percent), pharyngitis (30 percent), cough (28 percent), and conjunctivitis (17 percent) (Sharp et al., 1995). The incubation period ranges from two to seven days, after which fever appears rapidly, along with the other findings noted above. Joint and bone pain are also prevalent. There is generally a rash during the first few days of illness, followed by anorexia, nausea, vomiting and frequently respiratory manifestations that mimic a cold or flu. The fever usually breaks after three to six days, followed by a maculopapular or morbilliform rash on the trunk, spreading to the limbs and face and resolving after a few days. Patients then recover over several weeks although the convalescent period may extend a few more weeks. Dengue does not cause persistent or recurrent musculoskeletal complaints or arthritis (Monath, 1995).

Dengue hemorrhagic fever is the most serious manifestation of the disease. This process, an immunologic reaction, occurs for the most part in individuals already sensitized to the disease, either actively through infection or passively in infants through placental transfer of immunoglobulin from mother to child.

Initially, dengue hemorrhagic fever appears the same as dengue but after several days the patient deteriorates with prostration, restlessness, signs of circulatory collapse (diaphoresis, cold extremities, dyspnea, circumoral and peripheral cyanosis, and hemorrhagic manifestations). Available laboratory tests cannot identify who will ultimately develop this manifestation.

Diagnosis

Because the clinical presentation of dengue is not distinguishable from other infectious diseases, the diagnosis is made by laboratory testing. Laboratory tests available include isolation of the virus, demonstrating the presence of the viral antigen using immunoassay tests, or amplification of the viral nucleic acids using the polymerase chain reaction process (Sudiro et al., 1997). Patient sera can be used to test for the presence of anti-dengue virus antibody; demonstrating a significant increase in the antibody titer between the acute and convalescent sera confirms the infection. This has been an effective way to study exposure of U.S. troops deployed to areas where dengue is endemic (Sharp et al., 1995).

Treatment and Prevention

Dengue is treated by managing the patient's symptoms, rather than a specific treatment such as an antiviral agent. Patients suspected of infection should ensure that they are safe from additional mosquito bites.

No vaccines currently available protect against dengue, although several are undergoing investigation. The Centers for Disease Control and Prevention predicts that an effective vaccine will be available within the next decade.

Correlation with Gulf War Illnesses

Although some of the clinical findings of individuals with Gulf War illnesses have some minor similarities to the presenting findings of dengue, this infection does not cause chronic disease. Furthermore, laboratory testing is available to detect infection with dengue virus. No evidence of incident cases of dengue fever was found among those who served in the Gulf War (Richards et al., 1991).

Summary

Dengue and dengue hemorrhagic fever represent an important infection in tropical areas. The virus is spread through mosquitoes, manifests itself by non-specific findings, and has no specific treatment once the cause is identified. A chronic state of this viral infection is not known, and laboratory tests are readily available to detect infection. Increased antibody titers have not been observed in individuals who served in the Gulf War. Therefore, dengue is not a likely cause for unexplained chronic symptoms among Gulf War veterans.

SANDFLY FEVER

Introduction

Sandfly fever is also known as Phlebotomus fever, pappataci fever, and three-day fever. The disease is caused by the phleboviruses that are part of the Bunyaviridae family. There are at least five different phleboviruses, distinguished by their immunologic characteristics. Of these five types, two (Sicilian virus and Naples virus) are endemic in the Middle East. Infection with the virus causes a self-limited febrile illness.

During World War II, sandfly fever was a major problem for U.S. forces, with 19,000 cases reported (Oldfield et al., 1991). The highest incidence was in the Middle East, so military leaders were aware of the risk of sandfly fever during the Persian Gulf deployment. During World War II, attack rates were 3 to 10 percent of all troops, but among some units, the attack rate exceeded 50 percent. From a military standpoint, sandfly fever is a serious threat, since a large number of individuals can become infected and ill within a short period of time.

Epidemiologic Information

Sandfly fever is known to occur throughout the Middle East, the Mediterranean area, the Balkans, eastern Africa, and other neighboring areas. Most natives acquire the infection early in life and remain immune. The vector for this infection is the sandfly, *Phlebotomus papatasi*. Sandflies are small urban flies that are about 2 to 3 mm in size. Most patients (99 percent) who are bitten by the sandfly are unaware that they were bitten. The sandfly is the same vector responsible for transmitting *Leishmania* (Tesh, 1989).

The sandfly is primarily a nocturnal insect with the largest numbers appearing from April to October. (See the vector plots in Figure 6.1.) The female fly transmits the disease, starting about a week after she acquires the infection from an infected human host. The fly remains infected throughout life (about four more weeks). The gerbil may be a possible reservoir; however, the infected human is generally considered to be the primary host and source of infection for the sandfly.

What Infected Patients Experience

As one of its names implies, the illness associated with sandfly fever is of a short duration, generally on the order of two to four days. The incubation period is from three to six days, followed by a sudden onset of symptoms. Fever is usually the first, peaking sometimes as high as 105°F. Patients may experience severe frontal headaches, retroorbital pain, photophobia, arthralgias, and muscle aches. Nausea, vomiting, abdominal pain, and diarrhea may also occur. Some patients also have symptoms during infection that suggest an aseptic meningitis, at times sufficient to warrant evaluation of spinal fluid (Schwarz et al., 1995). After the initial three days, the fever gradually decreases. During convalescence, patients can experience giddiness, weakness, and depression

(Sanford, 1991). About 15 percent of patients experience a second attack between 2 and 12 weeks after the initial infection. Because of past experience, outcomes from this disease are well studied. Mortality is not observed.

Diagnosis

The infection can be made based on isolation of the virus starting just before fever onset and continuing for a day after onset. Serologic tests are also available for diagnosis of the infection.

Treatment and Prevention

Treatment is generally supportive in nature. Although some advocate ribavirin as a potential treatment, supportive care usually results in resolution of symptoms in a relatively short period of time.

Prevention centers on avoidance of sandfly bites. Spread can be prevented by using insecticides and mosquito nets to protect the infected individual from sustaining another bite, permitting subsequent transmission to an uninfected host. Further information can be found in the review of *Leishmania* by Oldfield and colleagues (1991).

Correlation with Gulf War Illnesses

No cases of sandfly fever were reported among Gulf War veterans, in contrast to the 30 cases of sandfly fever per 1,000 population (among those deployed to the Middle East) during World War II in the Persian Gulf region. The time of year when most troops were deployed during the Gulf War favored the low rate of *Leishmania* infection and the absence of sandfly fever. The prevalence of *P. papatasi* depends on environmental conditions; the sandfly is sensitive to temperature extremes and low humidity. Cross and colleagues (1996) used weather station and satellite data to model Persian Gulf weather conditions and predict the seasonal distribution of the sandfly. As diagrammed in Figure 6.1, the highest sandfly prevalence, and thus the highest risk of both *Leishmania* and sandfly fever, occurs in the spring and summer months. Laboratory studies among Gulf War veterans have failed to demonstrate any evidence of exposure to, or infection by, the sandfly fever virus (Richards et al., 1991).

Summary

Sandfly fever was a significant source of morbidity in previous military engagements. Protective measures, including mosquito nets and insecticides along with the timing of the operation, may have contributed to the lack of incident cases. A chronic state of this viral infection is not known, and laboratory tests are readily available to detect infection. Increased antibody titers have not been observed in individuals who served in the Gulf War. These combined findings suggest that sandfly fever is not a cause of the symptoms experienced by some individuals with Gulf War illnesses.

LEISHMANIAVIRUS

Introduction

Leishmaniavirus is a relatively recently recognized double-stranded RNA virus that infects some strains of *Leishmania*. This virus is a member of the family Totiviridae, a group of viruses that infect protozoa and fungi (Saiz et al., 1998). Viruses that infect protozoan parasites were first recognized in the 1960s; however, *Leishmania*-infecting viruses were discovered in 1988 (Chung et al., 1994). Although the molecular characteristics of this group of viruses have recently been elucidated, its relationship to clinical disease is essentially unknown. Leishmaniavirus has some unusual characteristics; specifically, a viral capsid protein is an RNA endonuclease that may be responsible for some of the viral persistence characteristics (MacBeth and Patterson, 1995). The virus has been detected in cultured *L. braziliensis*, *L. guyanensis*, and *L. major* (Saiz et al., 1998).

Epidemiologic Information

Little is known about this virus. However, in a study of human biopsy tissues collected in 1996 as part of a drug treatment program in Cuzco, Peru, viral RNA was identified in two of 11 samples studied by molecular diagnostic techniques (Saiz et al., 1998).

What Infected Patients Experience

Much more evaluation needs to be completed to understand whether infection of *Leishmania* with Leishmaniavirus alters the pathogenesis of the protozoa in humans. What clinical manifestations, if any, result from this infection would be speculative.

Diagnosis

The diagnosis of infection with Leishmaniavirus in patients who harbor a *Leishmania* infection is made through the use of molecular diagnostic techniques (Saiz et al., 1998). However, this diagnostic technique is currently performed only in specialized research laboratories.

Treatment and Prevention

Because this virus is present only in patients infected by *Leishmania*, the treatment and prevention are the same as those described in the discussion on *Leishmania*.

Correlation with Gulf War Illnesses

Because so little is known about this infection, correlation with unexplained Gulf War illnesses cannot be made at this time. However, because of the low rate of *Leishmania* among those who served in the Gulf War, it is unlikely that many, if any, veterans harbor this virus.

Summary

Leishmaniavirus is a newly described double-stranded RNA virus that has been found in some cases of *Leishmania* infections in Peru. Further research is needed to sufficiently understand the role of this virus in the pathogenesis of human disease. There is some speculation that the virus might modify the protozoan infection and influence the manifestations of disease in patients infected with *Leishmania*. At present, however, there is no evidence that a sufficient number of patients are infected with *Leishmania* that Leishmaniavirus could be present in more than, at most, a few individuals who served in the Gulf War.

Chapter Six

PARASITIC DISEASES

LEISHMANIASIS

Introduction

Leishmaniasis refers to a collection of clinical manifestations that are the result of a protozoal infection by members of the *Leishmania* family. Leishmaniasis generally does not spread from person to person; rather, infections are transmitted to people when they are bitten by an infected female sandfly. It is important to be aware of this infection because some of the symptoms found in infected patients are similar to those reported by some Gulf War veterans. Furthermore, a small number of Gulf War veterans have already been diagnosed as having leishmaniasis. Understanding what is known about infections with this organism, including the diseases it produces, can help put this infection in the overall context of the Gulf War illnesses. Although not all forms of leishmaniasis are known to exist in the Persian Gulf, this section begins with a discussion of leishmaniasis in general and then focuses on specific infections known to occur in the Middle East.

Leishmania is a microscopic parasite that can be seen only by trained professionals using a relatively high-powered microscope. The life cycle of the organism is interesting although not unique in nature. *Leishmania* are digenetic protozoa, meaning that they exist in two distinct life forms. *Leishmania* live in specific animal hosts (sometimes including humans) as aflagellar obligate intracellular amastigotes (2–3 μm in length) within mononuclear phagocytes. The organisms are transmitted from animal to animal (or animal to human) through an insect intermediate, particularly the sandfly, *Phlebotomus papatasi*, where *Leishmania* exist as flagellated, extracellular promastigotes (10–15 μm in length and 1.5–3.5 μm in width). To acquire the infection, the sandfly must first bite an infected animal (or person). Then the *Leishmania* organism transforms itself from the amastigote to the promastigote form in the sandfly. The infection is passed when the infected sandfly feeds on a new victim. From the standpoint of human disease, the usual animal host serves as the reservoir.

Different *Leishmania* species have traditionally been thought to cause different diseases, although they look the same when viewed under the microscope. The different species have been distinguished by the way they clinically affect their victims (hosts) and their geographic origin. Experts have recognized and classified the infections into four distinct clinical syndromes: cutaneous leishmaniasis, visceral leishmaniasis (known also as kala azar), mucocutaneous leishmaniasis, and diffuse cutaneous leishmaniasis. The first two are of interest to Gulf War veterans because the infectious organisms that cause these diseases exist in the Persian Gulf region.

Tables 6.1 and 6.2 show the common associations between cutaneous and visceral *Leishmania* infections, respectively, and the organisms that cause them.

Epidemiologic Information

Leishmaniasis is of interest in studying Gulf War illnesses because it is known to exist in the Persian Gulf region, because it causes a number of different symptoms, some of which are included in the Gulf War illnesses, and because leishmaniasis has been found in some Gulf War veterans. By early 1995, there were 12 cases of viscerotropic and 20 cases of cutaneous leishmaniasis diagnosed in U.S. troops who served in the Gulf War (Hyams et al., 1995). Cutaneous

Table 6.1

Old World Cutaneous Leishmaniasis

Organism	Geographic Areas	Animals Infected	Age/Gender Distribution	Incubation Period	Symptoms	Resolution
Leishmania tropica	Mediterranean Middle East India Southern Soviet Union	Humans and dogs	Urban children and younger adults	2–24 months	Single sore, usually on the face, slowly enlarges, crusty appearance	Heals over 1–2 years and scars, rarely spreads
Leishmania major	Middle East deserts Africa, Southern Soviet Union	Burrowing rodents and humans	All rural populations	2–8 weeks	Multiple sores, usually on legs, sometimes swollen lymph glands, moist appearance	Heals in 3–5 months with scarring

SOURCE: Locksley (1991). Reprinted by permission from *Harrison's Principles of Internal Medicine*, 12th ed., J.Wilson et al. (eds.), pp. 789–790, McGraw-Hill, New York, 1991. Copyright © 1991 McGraw-Hill, Inc.

NOTE: The cutaneous leishmaniasis types shown are the major ones associated with "old world cutaneous leishmaniasis." There are a number of "new world" types, but, since they are not likely to be relevant to those with Gulf War illnesses, they have not been included in this chart.

Table 6.2

Visceral Leishmaniasis

Organism	Subtype	Geographic Areas	Animals Infected	Age Distribution	Incubation Period	Symptoms	Resolution
Leishmania donovani	African	East Africa mostly	Dogs, other meat eating animals, humans	Ages 10–25	3 months (range 1–18 months)	Nighttime fevers, rapid heart rate, diarrhea, cough, liver problems, sometimes swollen lymph glands, anemia, and other blood problems	Requires treatment
	Mediterranean (a.k.a. *L. infantum*)	Mediterranean, China, Soviet countries	Dogs, jackals, foxes, humans, and probably rats	Infants usually; sometimes adults	Same as above	Same as above	Requires treatment
	Mediterranean (a.k.a. *L. chagasi*)	Latin America	Dogs, jackals, foxes, and humans	Infants usually; sometimes adults	Same as above	Same as above	Requires treatment
	Indian	India	Humans only	Ages 10–25	Same as above	Same as above	Requires treatment

SOURCE: Locksley (1991).

leishmaniasis was a known infectious disease problem for troops stationed in the Middle East during World War II, with an incidence of 1.93 cases per 1,000 population ("Unexplained illnesses among Desert Storm veterans . . . ," 1995; Cross and Hyams, 1996); therefore, it was anticipated that it might become a problem during the Gulf War. However, the incidence of leishmaniasis among Gulf War ground troops was only about 2–3 percent of that experienced in World War II.

What Infected Patients Experience

The specific symptoms experienced by infected individuals depend on the type of infection. Cutaneous and visceral disease are discussed separately.

Cutaneous Leishmaniasis. After infection, patients usually present with findings after two to eight weeks (the incubation period), although some cases have been reported following a one-year incubation period. The first is usually a reddish, inflamed swelling or lump that begins at the site of the sandfly bite. Over the next few months, the swelling grows until ultimately the skin opens in the form of an ulcer with a raised border and a crusty center. Because the sandfly generally bites its victim on exposed areas of the skin (e.g., face, extremities), these are the sites of most nodules and ulcers.

Classically, the organisms known to cause cutaneous leishmaniasis in the Middle East are *Leishmania tropica* and *Leishmania major*. Twenty cases of cutaneous leishmaniasis were diagnosed among Gulf War troops (Kreutzer et al., 1993). Among Gulf War troops, *L. major* was the cause of the cases of cutaneous leishmaniasis.

Visceral Leishmaniasis. Visceral leishmaniasis refers to the disseminated form of the disease; that is, patients with visceral leishmaniasis have an infection that involves multiple organs in the body. In its full-blown form, visceral leishmaniasis, known as kala azar, is a devastating disease with a high mortality rate. Visceral disease is classically associated with an infecting organism known as *Leishmania donovani*. Gulf War veterans, however, experienced the visceral form of the disease as a result of infection with *L. tropica*, a different species of *Leishmania* that is generally associated with the cutaneous form of the disease.

Most important, the visceral disease experienced by Gulf War troops appears to have been of a milder visceral form than that conventionally known. The disease is sufficiently different that it has been termed "viscerotropic" (meaning having an attraction to the body organs) leishmaniasis to distinguish it from classical visceral disease (Magill et al., 1993).

Magill described the findings found in the first eight patients; these are summarized in Table 6.3.

Two of these eight patients had other serious diseases; one was infected with HIV and another had a serious cancer of the kidney. The remaining six patients were otherwise healthy.

Table 6.3

**Findings Among First Eight Gulf War Veterans
Diagnosed with Viscerotropic Leishmaniasis**

Feature	Finding
Incubation period	1–14 months
Fever	5 of 8 patients
Abdominal pain	6 of 8 patients
Tiredness	7 of 8 patients
Fatigue	7 of 8 patients
Enlarged liver	4 of 8 patients
Enlarged spleen	4 of 8 patients

Diagnosis

Cutaneous leishmaniasis can be diagnosed histologically. The organisms appear in biopsy sections as round to oval bodies measuring from 2 to 4 μm without a capsule. The organisms are found within macrophages, sometimes up to

20 organisms within a single macrophage (Lever and Schaumburg-Lever, 1983). Culture is also an available diagnostic method that permits speciation of the parasite.

Diagnostic procedures for visceral leishmaniasis are considerably more invasive than those described for the cutaneous form. Because the organism resides in tissues, bone marrow aspirate and biopsy, lymph node biopsy, liver biopsy, and splenic biopsy are diagnostic options used in various countries (Locksley, 1991). Staining techniques similar to those described for the cutaneous form of the disease are then used to identify the organism. Current serologic assays (tests to look for evidence of infection using blood samples) are neither sensitive nor specific. Although new assays continue to be developed (Dillon et al., 1995), much additional research in this area is warranted to be able to better detect and understand the distribution of diseases caused by *Leishmania.*

Treatment and Prevention

Pentavalent antimonial compounds for three to four weeks are the first-line treatment drugs for patients with visceral leishmaniasis and for patients with the cutaneous form of disease when lesions are disfiguring or where mucocutaneous disease is prevalent. For patients with cutaneous disease that is not disfiguring, it is reasonable either to observe the patient or to treat with topical agents.

Most patients with visceral disease respond to treatment, although the rate of resistance to initial therapy, currently about 10 percent, is increasing. It is important, therefore, to ensure an accurate diagnosis before treatment and follow treatment guidelines explicitly.

Prevention centers on avoidance of sandfly bites. Spread can be prevented by using insecticides and mosquito nets to protect the infected individual from sustaining another bite, permitting subsequent transmission to an uninfected host. Further information can be found in the review of *Leishmania* by Oldfield and colleagues (1991).

Correlation with Gulf War Illnesses

Although it is possible that additional Gulf War veterans may have had viscerotropic leishmaniasis, the infection is unlikely to be present in a large population of Gulf War veterans. First, all patients who were identified with the disease were identified within just over a year following exposure. Second, the cutaneous disease, unlike the viscerotropic form, is easy to see and it is unlikely that more individuals would not have sought treatment if there was a major outbreak.

Leishmania is transmitted by the same vector, *Phlebotomus papatasi,* that causes sandfly fever. There were no cases of sandfly fever reported among Gulf War veterans, in contrast to the 30 cases of sandfly fever per 1,000 population (among those deployed to the Middle East) during World War II. The time of year when most troops were deployed during the Gulf War favored the low rate of *Leishmania* infection and the absence of sandfly fever. *Leishmania* must go through the promastigote stage in the sandfly, and a significant sandfly population exists in the region only during certain seasons. The prevalence of *P. papatasi* depends on environmental conditions; the sandfly is sensitive to temperature extremes and low humidity.

Cross and colleagues (1996) used weather station and satellite data to model Persian Gulf weather conditions and predict the seasonal distribution of the sandfly. Figure 6.1 shows the approximate results of the model and indicates that the highest sandfly prevalence, and thus the highest risk of both *Leishmania* and sandfly fever, occurs in the spring and summer months.

Because the sandfly is responsible for both the cutaneous and the viscerotropic form, a low rate of cutaneous disease suggests similar results for the more invasive form. Of the 12 patients identified with viscerotropic disease, only one was asymptomatic. Therefore, if the viscerotropic disease were more common, more patients with severe abdominal pain, fever, abnormal laboratory tests, and fatigue would be expected.

Similarly, although there is little experience with visceral disease caused by *L. tropica*, several of the patients studied extensively and reported by Magill et al. (1993) were not treated, and yet their disease resolved. This duration of illness and resolution is unlike that seen in kala azar, but it is similar to how the *L. tropica* organism behaves when it causes cutaneous disease.

There is no known evidence that *Leishmania* per se interacts with other infectious diseases or agents.[1] Like any other infectious agent, however, *Leishmania*

---

[1]Leishmaniavirus, recognized relatively recently (1988), is a double-stranded RNA virus that infects some strains of *Leishmania* (Chung et al., 1994). This virus is a member of the family Totiviridae, a group of viruses that infect protozoa and fungi (Saiz et al., 1998). Leishmaniavirus has some unusual characteristics; specifically, a viral capsid protein is an RNA endonuclease that may be responsible for some of the viral persistence characteristics (MacBeth and Patterson, 1995). The virus has been detected in cultured *L. braziliensis, L. b guyanensis,* and *L. major* (Saiz et al., 1998). Further research is needed to sufficiently understand the role of this virus in the pathogenesis of human disease. There is some speculation that the virus might modify the protozoan infection and influence the manifestations of disease in patients infected with *Leishmania.* At present, however, there is no evidence that sufficient patients are infected with *Leishmania* that Leishmaniavirus could be present in more than, at most, a few individuals who served in the Gulf War

RAND *MR1018/1-6.1*

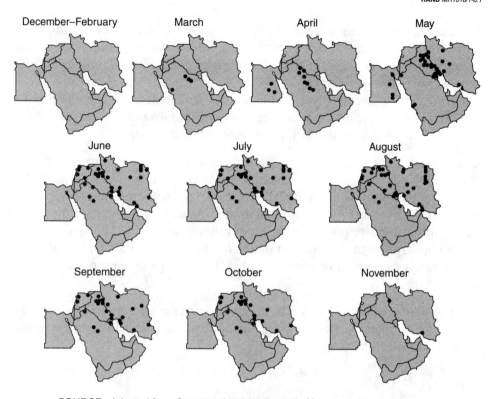

SOURCE: Adapted from Cross et al. (1996).Reprinted by permission from *American Journal of Tropical Medicine and Hygiene*, "Use of Weather Data and Remote Sensing to Predict the Seasonal Distribution of *Phlebotomus Papatasi* in Southwest Asia," 1996, Vol. 54, pp. 530–536. Copyright © 1991 American Society of Tropical Medicine and Hygiene.

Figure 6.1—Approximate Results of Model Show Predicted Sandfly Location by Month

interacts with the host's immune system. In fact, this interaction is responsible for much of the damage that occurs as a result of the infection. Some evidence suggests that a suppressed immune system, as occurs with AIDS and other diseases, can result in leishmaniasis taking on different manifestations. Immune system responses are covered in companion reports in this series, including the volume on stress (Marshall et al., 1999).

Review of the findings, particularly viscerotropic leishmaniasis, suggests that patients with leishmaniasis share some clinical symptoms (e.g., fatigue) with some patients with undiagnosed illnesses associated with Gulf War service. There has been considerable interest in those few Gulf War veterans known to be infected with this parasite.

Summary

Leishmania is important because infection is known to exist in the Middle East, military personnel and veterans are known to have become infected, and the symptoms resemble those of Gulf War illnesses. Presently, simple diagnostic tests for visceral and viscerotropic disease do not exist, although research to develop these tests is under way and should be accelerated. The finding of 12 cases of viscerotropic leishmaniasis caused by *L. tropica* reminds us that all the possible manifestations of infectious diseases are not known.

Leishmaniasis was a known infectious disease at the onset of Operation Desert Shield. Efforts to prevent exposure to the sandfly likely helped reduce the number of patients who ultimately became infected with the disease. Also, the timing of the operation was favorable in that the sandfly population increases during spring and summer months. Many military and civilian documents suggest a high level of understanding of where *Leishmania* exists and what steps can be taken to prevent or reduce it when U.S. troops are stationed in areas where it lives.

Because all of the known cases of leishmaniasis were diagnosed within just over a year after the Gulf War, it is unlikely that *Leishmania* is a major cause of unexplained Gulf War illnesses.

MALARIA

Introduction

Malaria in humans is caused by one of four plasmodia species that infect humans: *P. falciparum*, *P. vivax*, *P. ovale*, and *P. malariae*. Malaria has been recognized for over 3,500 years and is found primarily in Africa, Asia, South and Central America, and Oceania regions.

Seven cases of *P. vivax* were observed among individuals who served in the Gulf War. Malaria remains a serious problem, particularly in developing countries, with over 200 million cases and between one million and two million deaths annually. Malaria is also recognized as a particular problem for both military and civilian individuals who travel to areas where malaria is endemic.

Malaria is usually transmitted to humans through the bite of the infected female anopheline mosquito. Once they enter the body, the four species interact with the host somewhat differently. With all four, the sporozoite form present in mosquito saliva travels through the body to the liver. In the liver, they invade the liver cells (hepatocytes) and mature to become tissue schizonts (all four forms) or dormant hypnozoites (seen in *P. vivax* and *P. ovale*).

The schizonts produce thousands of merozoites (an amplification stage) after which they rupture the liver cell and are released into circulation to invade red blood cells. Within the red cells, the merozoites multiply, producing 24–32 offspring that, upon lysis of the red cell, continue the cycle by infecting subsequent erythrocytes. For *P. vivax* or *P. ovale*-infected individuals, hypnozoites can remain dormant for a number of months before they mature into schizonts, releasing merozoites into the blood and causing either a relapse or a delayed initial infection (most likely to occur in individuals taking prophylactic drugs during travel to endemic areas).

Within erythrocytes, some organisms develop into a gametocyte form (the sexual stage). The gametocytes enter the mosquito at the time of an insect bite, mature into gametes and then divide to produce the sporozoites. Sporozoites migrate to the mosquito salivary gland and then enter a new host upon a subsequent bite.

Patients may become infected through blood transfusion or through transmission during pregnancy. In these cases, there is not a relapsing course associated with *P. vivax* or *P. ovale* because no hypnozoite stage is established through initial hepatic infection.

Epidemiologic Information

P. falciparum occurs primarily in tropical areas throughout the world whereas *P. vivax* is common in tropical and temperate areas, *P. malariae* occurs worldwide, and *P. ovale* is less common with most cases identified in Western Africa, India, and South America. It is not surprising, therefore, that the seven patients with malaria were diagnosed with *P. vivax* infections. In more temperate areas where mosquitoes are prevalent only during summer months, the hypnozoite stage of *P. vivax* allows parasite survival in humans over the winter so that the infection can be again transmitted when the mosquito population increases in summer.

Among civilians in the United States (including foreigners and those of unknown origin), there were 151 cases of malaria in 1970, increasing to 1,838 in 1980 and dropping back to 976 in 1994 (Centers for Disease Control, 1997b).

What Infected Patients Experience

Fever cycles are the hallmark of malarial infection. Erythrocyte lysis with release of merozoites occurs usually just after a fever spike. The cycle frequency provides some insight into the type of malaria present. With *P. vivax* and *P. ovale*, cycles occur approximately every 48 hours whereas with *P. malariae* the cycle is 72 hours. Patients with *P. falciparum* infections usually experience on-going fevers with intermittent fever spikes. The cycle is characterized by a pro-dromal stage of several hours followed by a cold stage that can last minutes to hours and is often accompanied by shaking chills. Then the patient experiences the hot stage with a rapid fever rise around the time of schizont rupture. During these high fevers (up to or greater than 104°F), headache, hypotension, tachy-cardia, nausea, vomiting, diarrhea, and altered mental status are common. Several hours later the patient, who during the hot stage was relatively dry, en-ters a diaphoretic stage with profound sweating, defervescence, and fatigue.

By far the most dangerous form of malaria is the illness caused by *P. falciparum*. Only *P. falciparum* produces microvascular disease that results from adherence of the infected cells to endothelial cells of capillaries and small veins. This adherence blocks these vessels. Combined with other pathophysiologic effects, *P. falciparum* precipitates damage to essential organs, particularly the brain (cerebral malaria), kidney (renal failure), gastrointestinal tract (gastroenteritis), and lungs (pulmonary edema).

The other forms of malaria do not produce the microvascular disease observed with *P. falciparum*. *P. vivax* and *P. ovale* tend to infect younger erythroid cells (reticulocytes), therefore limiting the erythrocyte population they target. How-ever, as they lyse reticulocytes, these parasites stimulate increased red cell hematopoiesis, increasing the number of younger erythroid cells in the periph-eral blood.

Diagnosis

From the clinical standpoint, malaria should be included in the differential di-agnosis when a patient presents with fever in the presence of any risk factor for transmission, particularly travel to endemic areas. Diagnosis is established by finding parasites in Giemsa-stained blood films obtained from infected individ-uals. It may be necessary to draw several specimens to properly identify the or-ganism. Although some sensitive blood tests are available through the CDC, they are not routinely available in diagnostic laboratories, nor are they neces-sary to establish the diagnosis.

Treatment and Prevention

Treatment for malaria is well established, with cholorquine being the drug of choice for infections that are susceptible to this drug. Almost all cases of *P. vi-vax* are susceptible, although drug resistance can present a challenge to physi-cians treating patients infected with *P. falciparum*. Patients with resistant *P.*

vivax respond to other medications to eradicate the initial infection. Individuals infected with *P. vivax* and *P. ovale* are also treated with primaquine to obliterate the hypnozoites, preventing a relapse months after initial symptoms resolve ("Mefloquine and malaria prophylaxis," 1998; McCombie, 1996; Olliaro et al., 1996; White, 1997, 1998; Barat and Bloland, 1997).

A number of preventative strategies exist or are the subject of research. Current strategies include chemoprophylaxis for individuals traveling to endemic areas, vector control (mosquito abatement programs and insecticides), and use of re-pellants and mechanical barriers to mosquitoes. Vaccination is the subject of current research (Barron, 1998; Mills, 1998; Kain and Keystone, 1998; Kwiatkowski and Marsh, 1997; Kitua, 1997; Soares and Rodrigues, 1998; Connor et al., 1998; Greenwood, 1997; Facer and Tanner, 1997; Dubois and Pereira da Silva, 1995; Leo et al., 1994).

Correlation with Gulf War Illnesses

Because of the public health effect of malaria, infections with this organism are quite well understood. Regarding patients who returned to the United States with malaria, fewer than 5 percent of them became ill more than one year after arriving in the United States.

The known behavior of the *Plasmodium* species indicates that malaria is an ex-tremely unlikely etiology for unexplained Gulf War illnesses. All seven individ-uals who served in the Gulf War with malaria were diagnosed with *P. vivax*. Judging by clinical experience, very few patients initially present after one year. The constellation of symptoms included among those with unexplained Gulf War illnesses is inconsistent with what we know about malaria.

Summary

Malaria is known to exist in the Middle East, and a few military personnel and veterans were infected, experiencing classic malaria symptoms. Experienced laboratories should have no difficulty identifying the malaria parasite on com-monly used blood films, yet blood work on individuals with unexplained Gulf War illnesses has been repeatedly negative.

The clinical presentation of unexplained Gulf War illnesses is inconsistent with what we know about the clinical course of malaria. Almost all malaria cases manifest disease within the first year following exposure. The likelihood of persistent, subclinical disease is very remote.

GIARDIA

Introduction

Giardiasis is an illness caused by *Giardia lamblia* (also called *G. intestinalis* or *G. duodenalis*), a one-celled, microscopic parasite that lives in the intestines of people and animals. This parasite belongs to the family *Hexamitidae*. The organism is a flagellated enteric protozoa that is a common cause of morbidity throughout the world, including the United States. Primary findings in infected patients include diarrhea, abdominal cramps, bloating, and gas. Some estimate that *Giardia* accounts for up to 25 percent of North American gastroenteritis.

Giardia lamblia is a teardrop-shaped multiflagellar parasite that infects the upper small bowel of humans and other animals. This form of the organism is too fragile to survive outside the gut, but with normal bowel activity, *Giardia* transform and protect themselves in a membrane and undergo division to form cysts with four nuclei (Lujan et al., 1997). It is these cysts that are infective through the fecal-oral route. Cysts can survive in water for several months. Ingestion of 10 cysts can result in disease (Ortega and Adam, 1997). When in the gut, the parasite impairs absorption, particularly of fats and carbohydrates (Plorde, 1991b). As the organism populates the small intestine, it produces the clinical manifestations associated with giardiasis.

Epidemiologic Information

Giardia is ubiquitous. Random evaluation of stool suggests that there is a prevalence of about 4 percent in the United States (Hill, 1995). In other countries, the prevalence may exceed 20 percent (Plorde, 1991b). The most frequent source of infection is ingestion of contaminated water; drinking or swimming in unfiltered surface fresh water constitutes a potential risk as does travel to foreign countries with impure water and food supplies. Person-to-person transmission is the second most common source of infection, particularly for children in day care centers (especially if diapering is done), those caring for children in these centers, homosexual males, and institutionalized individuals (Hill, 1995; Thompson, 1994).

What Infected Patients Experience

The incubation period is typically one week, and the disease generally lasts 1–2 weeks, although a much longer duration, even years, is possible. The principal symptom is diarrhea (89 percent); other common findings include malaise (84 percent), flatulence (74 percent), foul smelling greasy stools (72 percent), abdominal cramps (70 percent), bloating (69 percent), nausea (68 percent), anorexia (64 percent), and weight loss (64 percent) (Hill, 1995). Not all patients will be symptomatic; however, asymptomatic patients can still pass infective cysts.[2] Stool examination for cysts at the time of symptom onset may be negative. In some patients, disease may persist for months with significant morbidity related to malabsorption and weight loss. The illness usually resolves after 1–4 weeks, although some patients develop an intermittent chronic infection with flatulence, abdominal pain, and soft stools.

Diagnosis

The standard for diagnosis of *Giardia* remains the identification of cysts or trophozoites in fecal material (Plorde, 1991b; Hill, 1995; Cook, 1995). As indicated, during the initial symptomatic phase organisms may not be identifiable in the stool. An alternative is the string test (Enterotest), whereby a nylon string or gastric tube is inserted through the mouth into the duodenum to sample contents. Serologic tests and other sensitive methods are also available to help the physician make the diagnosis of, and research the international distribution of, *Giardia*.

Treatment and Prevention

Prevention focuses on decreasing exposure to potentially infected water supplies and exercising caution when handling possibly infected body fluids. Individuals should, consistent with good general hygiene, wash hands after using the bathroom, after handling diapers, and before fixing food or drink. Individuals who are camping or traveling in foreign lands should avoid drinking improperly treated water. Water should be boiled for 10 minutes, chlorinated, or iodinated when uncertainty exists. Generally, municipal water supplies are considered safe. Swimming pools can be a source of infection; therefore, children with diarrhea should not swim.

A number of drugs are available for the treatment of giardiasis (Zaat et al., 1997). The dosing strategies (single dose, multiple doses over several days) vary depending on the drug and the patient population. In addition to specific antimicrobial therapy, supportive care in terms of fluid and electrolyte replacement is important. During treatment, household and sexual contacts should be examined and treated, even if asymptomatic, to prevent reinfection.

---

[2]CDC website: http://www.cdc.gov/ncidod/dpd/giardias.htm.

Correlation with Gulf War Illnesses

The clinical findings associated with giardiasis have been discussed. Because *Giardia* is a common infection, it is not surprising that some individuals who served in the Gulf War may have been, or currently are, infected with this parasite. However, the most common finding, namely, self-limited gastrointestinal disease, is not consistent with the long-term manifestations expressed by those individuals with undiagnosed Gulf War illnesses.

Summary

Giardia is a parasite that infects individuals either through the consumption of infected water or food or through person-to-person contact. The disease is usually self-limited, over a period of weeks, with the major complaints being gastrointestinal discomfort and diarrhea. Reliable diagnostic tests currently exist to aid in the diagnosis of this disease, the standard being demonstration of the organism in stool or duodenal contents. Although a number of Gulf War veterans are likely to have *Giardia* because it is ubiquitous, the clinical manifestations of this disease are not consistent with most medical complaints expressed by individuals with undiagnosed Gulf War illnesses.

AMOEBA

Introduction

Amebiasis is a disease of the large intestine caused by a one-celled parasite called *Entamoeba histolytica*. This parasite is found in the United States and around the world. In most infected individuals, the disease is asymptomatic, although there is spectrum of presentation, ranging from mild diarrhea to life-threatening dysentery. A number of species of amoeba naturally parasitize humans, but it is *E. histolytica* that is important in disease. Some individuals, particularly those who are immunosuppressed (e.g., on steroids, HIV infected, suffering from malnutrition), are at high risk of developing serious disease.

E. histolytica is a protozoa that is within the family *Entamoebidae*. The organism has a fairly simple life cycle. It exists in two forms—the mobile trophozoite and the cyst form. The trophozoite form is the one responsible for disease and lives either within the colon or in the wall of the colon (responsible for disease), living on bacteria and other material within the gut. When diarrhea occurs, the trophozoite can be seen in liquid stool by trained observers. Under usual circumstances, however, the organism usually encysts before it leaves the GI tract. The cysts can survive for weeks in moist environments whereas trophozoites die rapidly. The organism is passed from person to person through ingestion of cysts from contaminated water or produce, or via direct fecal-oral spread.

Epidemiologic Information

Man is the principal host for amebiasis although the organism can occasionally infect animals. The source of infection is the cyst that enters the stool in asymptomatic patients. Therefore, this infection is most prevalent where living conditions and socioeconomic factors favor its transmission. The disease is most common in impoverished areas, when knowledge of disease transmission is absent, and among individuals who are mentally impaired. The main predisposing factor is poor sanitation resulting in either direct fecal-oral spread or through ingestion of contaminated water or food. There are estimates that half of individuals in developing countries are infected, compared with about a 1–4 percent infection rate in the United States as a whole and a worldwide infection rate of about 10 percent (Plorde, 1991a; Ravdin, 1995). In the United States, the disease is most often seen in immigrants from developing countries, in homosexual men, particularly those who engage in anal-oral sex, and in those living in unclean domiciles.

What Infected Patients Experience

For the most part, individuals infected with *E. histolytica* are either asymptomatic or develop only mild intestinal symptoms, including abdominal tenderness or discomfort, loose or watery stools, and stomach cramping. These clinical findings are not unique to *E. histolytica*; other infections cause similar clinical presentations. Even though most strains are not invasive, treatment of all infected individuals is warranted.

Among symptomatic patients, the range of disease extends from intermittent diarrhea to fulminant dysentery. *E. histolytica* has a lytic effect on tissue, the reason for its name. Diarrhea may be intermittent (for months to years) with up to four loose or watery stools per day. Diarrhea is described as foul smelling and is accompanied with frequent abdominal cramps and bowel gas.

Fulminant disease can occur at any time or can be associated with an outbreak of water contamination, although it usually occurs randomly in those at highest risk of disease. For these unfortunate individuals, the onset may be abrupt with high fever (up to 104°F to 105°F), severe cramps, and bloody diarrhea. In other patients, onset may be more gradual, with increasing symptoms over a one- to three-week period. Abdominal tenderness, including hepatomegaly and hepatic tenderness, are frequently seen. It is in these patients that examination of the watery stool for trophozoites is beneficial. If diarrhea is severe, the patient should be evaluated for electrolyte imbalance. At the extreme, there may be transmural ulceration of the colon with hemorrhage or perforation, resulting in peritonitis. Less commonly, the organism may be found in other tissues, producing liver, lung, or brain abscesses (Charoenratanakul, 1997; Fujihara et al., 1996; Schumacher et al., 1995). Although some have thought *E. histolytica* infection to be responsible for irritable bowel syndrome (IBS), studies now suggest that this infection is not responsible for that condition (Sinha et al., 1997).

Diagnosis

Entamoeba histolytica must be differentiated from other intestinal protozoa. Distinction from the nonpathogenic *E. coli, E. hartmanni, E. polecki, E. gingivalis, Endolimax nana,* and *Iodamoeba bütschlii,* and from the possibly pathogenic *Dientamoeba fragilis* is possible (but not always easy) based on morphologic characteristics of the cysts and trophozoites. *Entamoeba dispar,* however, is morphologically identical to *E. histolytica,* and differentiation must be based on isoenzymatic, immunologic, or molecular analysis. Microscopic identification of trophozoites and cysts in the stool is the common method for diagnosing *E. histolytica* either in fresh stool or stool concentrates. Trophozoites can also be seen in aspirates and biopsy samples submitted to the surgical pathology laboratory.

Immunologic methods exist to identify infection. These techniques are most useful for diagnosing extraintestinal disease where stool examination is not rewarding. Antibody detection kits including indirect hemagglutination, enzyme immunoassay, and immunodiffusion are available commercially. Antigen detection measures are useful to aid the microscopic identification of organisms (Haque et al., 1998; Gonzalez-Ruiz et al., 1994).[3]

Treatment and Prevention

Treatment includes both supportive measures as well as medications specifically aimed at eliminating the infection. Supportive treatment includes replacement of fluids, electrolytes, and blood, as needed. Antiprotozoal medications are effective in combination, as some are more effective against infection in the intestine and others are more effective against tissue organisms. Drugs include iodoqinol, paromomycin, diloxanide furoate, and metronidazole.

The mainstay of prevention involves good sanitation and education of those individuals who are at highest risk for infection. Proper food handling, hand

---

[3]See also the CDC website: http://www.dpd.cdc.gov/dpdx/HTML/Amebiasis.htm.

washing, and avoiding potentially contaminated water and food are important. For individuals traveling to areas where there is increased risk of infection, agents exist for treatment of water to kill the infection.

Correlation with Gulf War Illnesses

The clinical conditions associated with amebiasis are not the common presenting complaints reported by individuals with undiagnosed Gulf War illnesses, although some of these individuals do have abdominal pain. It is possible, if not likely, that some individuals who served in the Gulf War will have amebiasis given that the infection is common in the United States as well as in most other parts of the world. However, good diagnostic tests for this infection exist; therefore, amebiasis is not a likely candidate to explain the undiagnosed illnesses reported by Gulf War veterans.

Summary

Amebiasis is caused by infection with the protozoa *Entamoeba histolytica*. In most individuals, infection is either asymptomatic or produces mild intestinal discomfort. A minority of patients experience serious disease that can include bloody diarrhea and lung, liver, or brain abscesses. The clinical picture is not consistent with undiagnosed Gulf War illnesses.

SCHISTOSOMIASIS

Introduction

Schistosomiasis, also known as bilharzia, is caused by parasitic worms (trematodes). Infection with *S. mansoni*, *S. haematobium*, and *S. japonicum* cause the majority of illnesses in humans. *S. haematobium* causes urinary schistosomiasis, *S. mansoni* causes intestinal schistosomiasis, and *S. japonicum* causes Asiatic intestinal schistosomiasis. Man is the only important definitive host for the first two species; wild and domestic animals are important reservoirs for the latter. Two other species, *S. mekongi* and *S. intercalatum*, are other important members of this group that cause human disease. Although schistosomiasis is not found in the United States, 200 million people are infected worldwide, second only to malaria in terms of worldwide morbidity and mortality (McCully et al., 1976). The adult worms measure about 1–2 cm in length and live in the venous system of the intestine or urinary bladder.

What is unique to these and other worms is their life cycle. All of these organisms require passage through the snail (*Biomphalaria* sp. for *S. mansoni*, *Bulinus* sp. for *S. haematobium*, and *Oncomelania* sp. for *S. japonicum*) in water to become infective. They are not passed directly from person to person. The human host releases eggs through the urine or feces into water. In the water, the eggs hatch into the ciliated motile miracidia form that quickly penetrates the body of the snail intermediate host. Inside the snail, the miracidia multiply asexually, and after a period of about 4–6 weeks hundreds of infective motile cercariae emerge. In this form they have a forked tail and the ability to penetrate intact human skin, in part because they release digestive enzymes to facilitate their passage. People wading, swimming, bathing, or washing in contaminated fresh water are at risk. At penetration, the forked tail drops off and the cercaria becomes a schistosomule. This form then migrates into a vessel where it is transported to the lungs and ultimately to the liver. The worms then become sexually mature in the liver venules of man and migrate to their final, species-specific location. Here the worms can live many years and produce eggs that then repeat the above cycle.

Epidemiologic Information

Schistosomiasis is present in many parts of the world, including Africa, Latin America, the Caribbean, the Middle East (Iran, Iraq, Saudi Arabia, Syrian Arab Republic, Yemen), Southern China, and Southeast Asia.

S. haematobium and S. mansoni are both endemic in the Middle East. Historically, the Nile basin is probably the origin of S. haematobium and the African lake plateau the source of S. mansoni (McCully et al., 1976). It is important to remember, however, that human infection requires a body of fresh water in which the intermediate host snail lives.

What Infected Patients Experience

Shortly after infection, the patient may develop a papular rash or cutaneous irritation (schistosome dermatitis), sometimes known as swimmer's itch. However, most people have no symptoms at this early phase of infection.

The next phase is that of acute schistosomiasis, also known as Katayama fever (rare in S. haematobium infection). The patient exhibits fever, chills, cough, asthma, hives, dysentery, weakness, weight loss, abdominal pain, and muscle aches that generally begins two to six weeks following infection (McCully et al., 1976; Rabello, 1995).[4] The acute symptoms, associated with initial egg deposition, diminish over time but may last for several months. Symptoms of schisto-

---

[4]CDC website: http://www.cdc.gov/ncidod/dpd/schisto.htm.

somiasis are caused by the body's reaction to the eggs produced by worms, not by the worms themselves.

Rarely, eggs are found in the brain or spinal cord and can cause seizures, paralysis, or spinal cord inflammation (Pittella, 1997). Long-term complications from infection can result in damage to the infected organs, including the liver, intestines, lungs, and bladder (Shekhar, 1994; Strickland, 1994; Butterworth et al, 1994, 1996; "Infection with schistosomes . . . ," 1994; Helling-Geis et al., 1996; Hagan, 1996; Morris and Knauer, 1997). Even without treatment, damage to these organs occurs only rarely.

Most patients do well, but there is significant morbidity associated with schistosome infections. The development of periportal fibrosis or portal hypertension can develop over time. Although immunologically mediated, the specifics of this process are not well understood (Cheever, 1997). When studied in patients infected with *S. mansoni*, this process develops over many years. Hepatic function is generally acceptable; patients present with hematemesis or splenomegaly from the portal hypertension. Despite these findings, some patients tend to do better than others with portal hypertension (e.g., alcoholics). In patients infected with *S. mansoni* who develop portal hypertension, glomerulonephritis and cor pulmonale can result in increased morbidity (Nash, 1991).

Diagnosis

Because the geographic distribution of this infection is well known, diagnosis starts with a history, looking for travel to endemic areas and exposure to water sources that may be contaminated (Ruff, 1994). The definitive diagnosis is made through examination of feces or urine for the presence of schistosome eggs (Elliott, 1996). A blood test has been developed and is available through the Centers for Disease Control and Prevention[5]; however, the blood must be collected at least 6–8 weeks following exposure to provide adequate sensitivity

Treatment and Prevention

Effective and safe drugs are available for the treatment of schistosomiasis (Shekhar, 1994; Elliott, 1996; Brindley, 1994), including praziquantel, which is a broad-spectrum antihelminthic agent. These drugs are usually taken for one or two days, depending on the specific infection.

To prevent infection, individuals should avoid swimming or wading in fresh water in countries where schistosomiasis is endemic. Swimming in the ocean

---

[5]CDC website: http://www.cdc.gov/ncidod/dpd/schisto.htm.

and in chlorinated swimming pools is generally thought to be safe. Travelers should avoid drinking contaminated water. Water coming directly from canals, lakes, rivers, streams, or springs should be boiled for one minute or filtered before drinking. Iodine alone is insufficient to eliminate all parasite risk.

Bath water should be heated for five minutes to 150°F. Water held in a storage tank for at least 48 hours should be safe for showering. Vigorous towel drying after an accidental, brief water exposure may help to prevent the *Schistosoma* parasite from penetrating the skin. However, the CDC notes that this may not prevent infection.[6]

Correlation with Gulf War Illnesses

The clinical manifestations and the duration of illness associated with schistosomiasis are quite different from the findings reported among veterans with undiagnosed Gulf War illnesses. Furthermore, although troops were in the Persian Gulf, infection with schistosomiasis requires contact with bodies of fresh water with the intermediate host snails. Only a small number of individuals entered Iraq near the Euphrates River valley, where exposure to schistosomiasis may have occurred (Lashof et al., 1996).

Summary

Schistosomiasis is caused by infection with a member of the genus *Schistosoma*. Five different species commonly cause human disease. Schistosomiasis has a complex life cycle that requires an intermediate stage in a specific snail intermediate host. These snails live in fresh water; therefore, human infection can occur only when an individual is exposed to infected water where the snail and the trematode are endemic. Because of the requirement for bodies of fresh water and the difference between the clinical presentation of schistosomiasis and individuals with Gulf War illnesses, this infection cannot be the etiology for symptoms veterans are experiencing.

---

[6]CDC website: http://www.cdc.gov/ncidod/dpd/schisto.htm.

Chapter Seven

BIOLOGICAL WARFARE AGENTS

Biological warfare agents were one of the most feared classes of weapons that coalition troops believed Iraq might use against them. Biologic agents can either be sufficiently toxic that they kill their victims quickly, or they may induce a sufficient degree of acute disability that troops cannot fight effectively or defend themselves against an attack. The Centers for Disease Control and Prevention (2000) recently reviewed aspects of biological and chemical terrorism, looking at likely threats, particularly although not exclusively at civilian vulnerability. Although a number of possible biological warfare agents are known, the ones considered most likely to be used against Gulf War troops were anthrax and botulinum toxin. The medical consequences of exposure to these two agents[1] are well understood (Iowa Persian Gulf Study Group, 1994), and diagnosis, treatment, and prevention strategies exist for each.

ANTHRAX

Introduction

Among the known pathogenic bacteria, *Bacillus anthracis*, the causative agent of anthrax, is among the most feared. As a biologic warfare agent, *B. anthracis* is likely to be disseminated through the air (an aerosol). *B. anthracis* causes disease primarily in plant-eating animals; however, it does infect humans when they come in close contact with infected animals or animal products. The importance of anthrax has been recognized for years; in fact, the first description is found in the book of Genesis. Considered the fifth plague in 1491 BC, the infection was noted for killing Egyptian cattle. During the last century, the number of cases reported in developed countries has decreased.

---

[1]This report deals only with Anthrax and botulism toxin. Other biological weapon agents exist but were not known to be in the Gulf. Toxins that could be classed as either biological weapon or chemical weapon agents are dealt with in a companion report (Augerson, 2000).

What Infected Patients Experience

Naturally acquired disease typically occurs in one of three types—cutaneous anthrax, respiratory anthrax, or gastrointestinal anthrax. In developed countries, most anthrax cases are of the skin or "cutaneous" type (95 percent); approximately 5 percent are of the respiratory type. The cutaneous type ultimately causes ulceration and scarring over a several-week period, although about 20 percent of untreated cases result in death. The respiratory form has a much higher mortality, being usually fatal. This is the type of infection expected with use of *B. anthracis* as a biological warfare agent.

Respiratory anthrax is contracted by breathing in bacterial spores, as would be the case when *B. anthracis* is used as a biological warfare agent. This type of anthrax has two phases. The first phase occurs with a relatively small exposure (e.g., animal contact) and is sometimes nondescript with patients manifesting symptoms similar to the common cold or flu (e.g., tiredness, muscle aches, mild fever, and a nonproductive cough). Some patients also experience some chest tightness. At this stage, physical examination is not revealing, and diagnosis is difficult. After several days patients improve, again leading the patient and physician to attribute the symptoms to a cold or flu. Shortly thereafter patients experience the sudden onset of respiratory symptoms including shortness of breath and inability to take in oxygen. Patients usually die (from pulmonary hemorrhage) within 24 hours of the onset of this phase of the disease.

Prevention

Vaccination[2] is effective (92.5 percent) in preventing anthrax infection (Lew, 1995), which is why some individuals (approximately 150,000) deployed to the highest-risk areas of the Persian Gulf were vaccinated against anthrax. Although the initial findings in patients infected with anthrax mimic some of the findings in individuals with Gulf War illnesses, anthrax is not known to have a chronic state. Therefore, its use as a biologic warfare agent would have resulted in the devastating findings discussed above in multiple individuals shortly after exposure.

BOTULINUM TOXIN

Introduction

Clostridium botulinum is the pathogenic bacterium that is the causative agent of botulism. However, unlike *B. anthracis*, it is not the bacterium itself that is

---

[2]For a complete discussion of vaccine, see the companion report in this series (Golomb, forthcoming).

toxic but rather the toxins produced by the bacteria. These toxins affect the nervous system, resulting in weakness. Although tetanus results from toxins produced by another member of the same family of bacteria (*Clostridium tetani*), tetanus toxin acts on a different part of the nervous system and produces muscle spasm and rigidity (Bleck, 1995).

Epidemiologic Information

Before modern medicine, the botulism fatality rate was over 60 percent; however, with current medical intervention the overall fatality rate is less than 10 percent. Because botulism carries a high morbidity and mortality, it is considered a biological warfare agent (Wiener, 1996). Depending on the strain, *C. botulinum* produces different toxins, designated A through G, of which types A, B, E, and F cause human disease (Townes et al., 1996; Inoue et al., 1996; Jean et al., 1995; Singh et al., 1995; Weber et al., 1993). This bacterium is found throughout the world and can survive in harsh conditions.

What Infected Patients Experience

The toxin may ingested with food or water and absorbed into the blood and then progress via the blood to the nervous system. There is also wound botulism, where the infection begins at an open wound where bacteria grow and produce the toxin. Botulinum toxin can also be delivered by the aerosol route; this method affords broader area spread, greater casualties, and less loss of the agent than introducing it into the food or water supplies. Because toxins are environmentally stable, this is the most probable route to deliver this agent as a biological weapon. The presence of the toxin, however, determines the clinical manifestations, rather than how or where the toxin enters the body. The chemical structure and mechanism of action for each of the seven toxins is similar. The toxin cleaves at least one of three proteins that are involved in bringing the neurotransmitter acetylcholine to the nerve synapse (the location where the nerve to nerve transmission of information occurs). Cleavage by the neurotoxin inhibits acetylcholine release from the synapse (Schiavo and Montecucco, 1997). With the loss of communication between nerves, paralysis results.

The dominant clinical features of botulism are the neurologic symptoms secondary to toxin-mediated blockade of the voluntary motor and autonomic cholinergic junctions (Centers for Disease Control and Prevention, 1998). With mild botulism, patients may experience only dry mouth, inability to focus (perceived as blurred vision), and diplopia. With more severe disease, dysphonia, dysarthria, dysphagia, and peripheral muscle weakness may ensue. When the respiratory system fails, mechanical ventilator support becomes necessary, often for many weeks. The recovery period reflects the time for the body to re-generate damaged nerve fibers.

Like anthrax, chronic states of botulism are not known. If there had been a significant exposure to botulinum toxin during the Gulf War, the severe, dis-abling, and life-threatening findings discussed above would have been seen at that time. Although a low-level exposure has been hypothesized, this does not appear to be the case for these agents. Recently, this toxin has been used in low doses to successfully treat patients who have conditions associated with in-creased muscular activity (e.g., twitching and spasm) (Joo et al., 1996; Rebolleda and Munoz Negrete, 1996; Richman, 1997; Sampaio et al., 1997; Esper et al., 1997; Sood et al., 1996; Behari and Raju, 1996). To date, symptoms similar to Gulf War illnesses have not been reported in patients receiving therapeutic doses of botulinum toxin.

SUMMARY

Both anthrax and botulinum toxin result in recognizable, characteristic symp-toms that can be confirmed by available diagnostic techniques. No cases were diagnosed, and it is therefore highly unlikely that any exposure occurred.

Chapter Eight

UNIDENTIFIED INFECTIONS

For known infectious agents, the spectrum of disease they cause is fairly well characterized. That is not to say that infectious agents cannot emerge or change, manifesting different signs and symptoms over time. The signs and symptoms caused by the biologic warfare agents discussed, for example, are well known. Because these agents do not cause low-level chronic disease, they are unlikely to cause symptoms that have been associated with illnesses among Gulf War veterans.

Is it possible that new presently unidentified infectious diseases might account for the spectrum of disease associated with illnesses among Gulf War veterans? Such a possibility cannot be dismissed even though, based on past history, such a finding would be unlikely. For example, HIV, responsible for AIDS, and *Ileli-cobacter pylori*, responsible for gastrointestinal ulcers, were unknown when the diseases associated with them were first described. As discussed above, however, these diseases presented with definitive and verifiable clinical findings such as unusual infections and unexpected cancers with AIDS, and ulceration on endoscopy with *H. pylori*.

GENERAL PROCESSES FOR IDENTIFICATION

Investigational techniques center on trying to identify new agents when illnesses are discovered that might be infectious but for which a known cause is absent. When looking for agents, some issues include whether the presentation is acute or chronic and whether a case definition (well-defined conditions associated with specific illnesses) exists. With respect to the poorly defined illnesses associated with Gulf War service (a problematic case definition by the above criteria), many individuals deployed to the Gulf report that they do not feel as well on return as they did before they left.

How should one go about looking for differences between Gulf War veterans who are ill and those who are not? The case-control study approach is the proper epidemiologic technique. However, conducting these studies now is difficult because patients have been out of service for almost a decade. Physicians and other scientists look for evidence of exposure to infectious agents by comparing levels of antibodies in the blood before an illness to levels after recovery. In a similar way, it might be possible to compare blood serum samples from veterans that were collected before deployment with samples drawn on these same individuals after their return. If the differences in these "pre-post" sample comparisons are significantly bigger in those deployed to the Persian Gulf than in those who were not, then an epidemiologic difference exists that might explain causality.

To look for unknown agents, a number of relatively new approaches and techniques are being taken.

REPRESENTATIONAL DIFFERENCE ANALYSIS (RDA)

This technique amplifies the genetic information (DNA) present in specimens of patient's tissues (in the case of illnesses among Gulf War veterans this would generally be blood—particularly white blood cells). Samples from patients with illnesses among Gulf War veterans and from those who do not have the illnesses are treated the same. Then investigators subtract the DNA that is common to both the patients and the healthy control volunteers. The remaining DNA must then be evaluated to determine its nature and whether it represents nuclear material from an unknown infectious agent. This technique was used to demonstrate the presence of herpes virus in samples of Kaposi's sarcoma, a malignancy found in some AIDS patients (Relman, 1997; Fredericks and Relman, 1996; Lisitsyn, 1995; Baldocchi and Flaherty, 1997).

SERIAL ANALYSIS OF GENOMIC EXPRESSION (SAGE)

This method has properties similar to that of RDA. Using this technique, the characteristics of an organism are identified or determined by the genetic information that it expresses (Velculescu et al., 1995). This method allows researchers to look simultaneously at a large number of genetic messages and to quantify the genetic information identified.

CDNA EXPRESSION ANALYSIS

This is another genetic technique that looks for evidence that messenger RNA (mRNA) is present in a sample. mRNA is the nuclear material that takes genetic messages from the nucleus of the cell and tells the cell what proteins to make. The technique looks at genes that have been characterized. One then uses this technique to look for differences in the types of mRNA expressed by patients and nonpatients. Once differences exist between patients and nonpatients, the differences may be characterized (Hayashi et al., 1995).

The techniques discussed can be considered emerging approaches, but they have been useful in beginning to look for unexplained causes of illness. Presently, they are being evaluated to search for causes of chronic fatigue syndrome, illnesses among Gulf War veterans, and other conditions.

Chapter Nine

CONCLUSIONS AND RECOMMENDATIONS

This report reviews infectious diseases from the standpoint of those infections or potential infections known or thought to be present in the Persian Gulf during the Gulf War. To highlight potential causes of illness in Gulf War veterans, the review documents that some veterans were exposed to infectious diseases. Some of these diseases are common and generally self-limited (e.g., gastroenteritis, mild respiratory infections). These infections were identified and routinely treated in the Gulf. Other infections have been detected in a small group of veterans (e.g., *Leishmania*); however, findings do not suggest that these infections are a common cause of undiagnosed illness among those who served in the Gulf War. *Leishmania* is challenging to diagnose and efforts to develop better diagnostic tests should continue to be encouraged.

There remains controversy about the extent to which *Mycoplasma* might contribute to illness experienced by veterans. Consequently, some specific recommendations exist with respect to further investigation into *Mycoplasma* as a possible etiology for some cases of illness among Gulf War veterans.

- Testing of nucleoprotein gene tracking should proceed as planned. Efforts should be made to standardize testing procedures across different institutions, emphasizing sensitive, specific, and reliable testing methods. Antibody testing should be compared to PCR (and perhaps nucleoprotein gene tracking) for sensitivity and abandoned if it is confirmed to have a low sensitivity.

- Further efforts should be made to evaluate ill PGW veterans and healthy controls for the presence of *Mycoplasma* using PCR (and possibly nucleoprotein gene tracking, pending results of reliability tests). At least one control group should consist of healthy nonveterans, since cofactors associated with development of illness, or latency to illness for *Mycoplasma*, are not well defined.

- Efforts should be made to quantitatively characterize symptom frequencies in ill Gulf War veterans who test positive for *Mycoplasma fermentans* (using PCR) and in those who test negative.

- Tests of treatment with antibiotics should be performed upon ill Gulf War veterans in whom PCR testing for *Mycoplasma* is positive, even though mycoplasma has not been confirmed as an etiology. There are few treatments available where existing evidence suggests benefit; therefore, it is particularly important that promising treatments be given careful consideration and controlled testing.[1]

- Thus, a randomized controlled double blind treatment trial of antibiotics, of adequate duration, would be useful in ill Gulf War veterans, following testing for *Mycoplasma* (with PCR) and for herpes-virus 6. Outcome measures should include symptoms, quality of life, and post-treatment *Mycoplasma* test results. At least one powered subset should consist of veterans who test positive for *Mycoplasma* and negative for herpes-virus 6. Even if *Mycoplasma* per se is not confirmed to be a source of illness, there is merit to such a treatment trial in the face of reports of marked benefit with antibiotic therapy.

---

[1] Since this writing, such a study is now under way with many of the characteristics advised here.

ADDITIONAL CONSIDERATION ON *MYCOPLASMA*

If *Mycoplasma* is a significant source of disease in ill Gulf War veterans, it is possible that coinfection with other organisms may complicate response to treatment. *Mycoplasma* genetic material has been reportedly identified more often in patients with CFIDS than in healthy controls (Choppa et al., 1998; Vojdani et al., 1998; Nasralla et al., 1999). (CFIDS is another condition with chronic debilitating symptoms, to which illness in Gulf War veterans has been compared.) However, other agents, such as herpes-virus 6, have also been reported by some to be elevated in CFIDS (although the relation of herpes-virus 6 to CFIDS has been called into question) (Bond, 1993; Gupta and Vayuvegula, 1991; Wahren and Linde, 1991; Moutschen et al., 1994). Consideration should be give to testing for herpes-virus 6 (and perhaps other hypothesized agents) as well as *Mycoplasma* before entry into *Mycoplasma* treatment trials. In the event that more than one agent promotes illness symptoms, then treatment of *Mycoplasma* could fail to produce resolution selectively (or more commonly) in individuals who test positive for other agents. Understanding this potential source of treatment response heterogeneity would be important for identifying subgroups who may have differential potential to receive benefit from treatment.

Other potential factors may complicate evaluation of *Mycoplasma* as a source of illness in Gulf War veterans. *Mycoplasma* "adhesins" have extensive sequence homology to mammalian structural proteins, and for decades it has been suggested that this mimicry may cause *Mycoplasma* to provoke an anti-self response that triggers immune disorders. *Mycoplasma* adhesins exhibit sequence homologies with human CD4 and class II major histocompatibility complex lymphocyte proteins, which could generate autoreactive antibodies and trigger cell killing and immunosuppression. *Mycoplasma*, through "superantigens" for instance, may serve as B-cell and T-cell mitogens (substances that promote splitting or "mitosis," and cell transformation, of B- and T-type lymphocytes) and induce autoimmune disease through activation of T-cells directed against self, or polyclonal B-cells (Joseph, 1997).[1] For instance, *Mycoplasma arthritidis* superantigen appears to induce a lymphokine profile that favors activation of B-cell function, which may heighten the risk of triggering autoimmune disease in rodents.[2] The multiorgan protean manifestations of mycoplasmal infections in humans are considered by some to be consistent with the pathogenesis of autoimmunity (Joseph, 1997).

If a bacteria-mediated autoimmune disorder is provoked, then disease could persist after the inciting infection abates or is eradicated. Supporting this possibility are results of studies producing experimental arthritis in rodents by introducing *Mycoplasma*. Organisms are readily cultured from the joints early but later become increasingly difficult to recover even in the presence of severe active inflammation.[3] Moreover, in the case of rheumatoid arthritis, treatment with antibiotics appears to be more effective early in the course of disease.[4] It would be instructive to determine whether isolation of *Mycoplasma* differs early and late in the course of illness in Gulf War veterans (although early disease may be rare almost a decade after the putative exposure). If *Mycoplasma* is a cause of illness in PGW veterans (and perhaps also if *Mycoplasma* is not), then response to treatment may be less successful with increasing time from onset of disease.

If there is merit to the hypothesis that cytokine shifts favoring a Th2 cytokine profile occur as a result of Gulf War exposures, as has been postulated, and if this results in heightened susceptibility to intracellular infections including *Mycoplasma* infections, then acquisition of *Mycoplasma* infection could have occurred at a higher rate in Gulf War veterans than in controls long after the cytokine-shifting "exposures" occurred in the Gulf War. By this hypothesis, acquisition of the *Mycoplasma* infection could occur *after* departure from the Gulf or from the service, although susceptibility to this infection might be conditioned by exposures in the Gulf War.

Although it must be emphasized that this is entirely speculative, in this scenario, it is not necessary to postulate vaccine contamination or any other means of increased *Mycoplasma* exposure in the Gulf War. Rather, similar *Mycoplasma* exposure (perhaps even associated with similar antibody responses) may be more likely to lead to *Mycoplasma* colonization or infection, and perhaps to "disease" in Gulf War veterans than in controls. Moreover, it is possible that Th2 cytokine shifts may be associated with illness that has nothing to do

---

[1] L. Millett, letter to Garth Nicolson (1996); K. Roberts, letter to Garth Nicolson (1996).

[2] R. Synder, letter to Garth Nicolson (1996).

[3] L. Millett, letter to Garth Nicolson (1996); R. Toth, letter to Garth Nicolson (1996).

[4] J. Baseman, personal communication to Beatrice Golomb (1997).

with *Mycoplasma*, but occurs through distinct mechanisms (infectious or otherwise). This hypothesis is an area for possible research.[5]

---

[5]Detectable *Mycoplasma* could merely represent an "innocent bystander" consequence of the cytokine shift. (This hypothesis predicts that *Mycoplasma*-negative, ill Gulf War veterans with Th2 cytokine shifts, presumably from other causes, would acquire future *Mycoplasma* infection at a higher rate than controls without such cytokine shifts, and that the rate of development of illness in Th2-shifted Gulf War veterans who are not currently ill would be independent of conversion to the *Mycoplasma* -positive state.)

Abuekteish F, Daoud AS, Massadeh H, Rawashdeh M. *Salmonella typhi* meningitis in infants. *Indian Pediatr.* 1996;33:1037–1040.

Al'Aldeen AA, Cartwright KA. *Neisseria meningitidis*: vaccines and vaccine candidates. *J Infect.* 1996;33:153–157.

Al-Arabi MA, Hyams KC, Mahgoub M, Al-Hag AA, el-Ghorab N. Non-A, non-B hepatitis in Omdurman, Sudan. *J Med Virol.* 1987;21:217–222.

al-Khonizy W, Reveille JD. The immunogenetics of the seronegative spondyloarthropathies. *Baillieres Clin Rheumatol.* 1998;12:567–588.

Al-Shammari SA, Nass M. Family practice in Saudi Arabia: chronic morbidity and quality of care. *Int J Qual Health Care.* 1996;8:303–308.

Alballa SR. Epidemiology of human brucellosis in southern Saudi Arabia. *J Trop Med Hyg.* 1995;98:185–189.

Alshawe A, Alkhateeb G. Test of Iraqi anthrax vaccine with other vaccines. *J Biol Sci Res.* 1987;17:1–16.

Altekruse SF, Stern NJ, Fields PI, Swerdlow DL. *Campylobacter jejuni*—an emerging foodborne pathogen. *Emerg Infect Dis.* 1999;5:28–35.

Alter MJ. Epidemiology of hepatitis C. *Hepatology.* 1997;26:62S–65S.

Alter MJ, Mast EE, Moyer LA, Margolis HS. Hepatitis C. *Infect Dis Clin North Am.* 1998;12:13–26.

Analysis of endemic meningococcal disease by serogroup and evaluation of chemoprophylaxis. *J Infect Dis.* 1976;134:201–204.

Apicella MA. *Neisseria Meningitidis.* In: Mandell GL, Bennett JE, Dolon R, eds. *Principles and Practice of Infectious Diseases.* Vol. 2. 5th ed. New York: Churchill Livingstone, Inc.; 2000:1896–1909.

Arthur R, El-Sharkawy M, Cope S, et al. Recurrence of Rift Valley fever in Egypt. *Lancet.* 1993;342:1149–1150.

Asa PB, Cao Y, Garry RF. Antibodies to squalene in Gulf War syndrome. *Experimental and Molecular Pathology.* 2000;68(1):55–64.

Augerson W. A *Review of the Scientific Literature As It Pertains to Gulf War Illnesses,* Vol. 5: *Chemical and Biological Warfare Agents.* Santa Monica, Calif.: RAND, MR-1018/5, 2000.

Baldocchi RA, Flaherty L. Isolation of genomic fragments from polymorphic regions by representational difference analysis. *Methods.* 1997;13:337–346.

Barat LM, Bloland PB. Drug resistance among malaria and other parasites. *Infect Dis Clin North Am.* 1997;11:969–987.

Barbuddhe SB, Yadava VK, Singh DK. Detection of IgM and IgG antibodies against *Brucella* by dot-ELISA in humans. *J Commun Dis.* 1994;26:1–5.

Barbuddhe SB, Yadava VK. Efficacy of indirect haemolysis test in the diagnosis of human brucellosis. *J Commun Dis.* 1997;29:283–285.

Barron BA. Chemoprophylaxis in US Naval aircrew transiting malaria endemic areas. *Aviat Space Environ Med.* 1998;69:656–665.

Baseman J, Tully J. *Mycoplasmas*: Sophisticated, reemerging, and burdened by their notoriety. *Emerging Infectious Diseases.* 1997;3:21–32.

Baseman JB, Lange M, Criscimagna NL, Giron JA, Thomas CA. Interplay between *mycoplasmas* and host target cells. *Microb Pathog.* 1995;19:105–116.

Baseman JB, Reddy SP, Dallo SF. Interplay between *mycoplasma* surface proteins, airway cells, and the protean manifestations of *mycoplasma*-mediated human infections. *Am J Respir Crit Care Med.* 1996;154:S137–S144.

Bassily S, Boctor FN, Farid Z, Fanous A, Yassin MY, Wallace CK. Acute hepatitis non-A non-B in Cairo residents (a preliminary report). *Trans R Soc Trop Med Hyg.* 1983;77:382–383.

Bean NH, Goulding JS, Lao C, Angulo FJ. Surveillance for foodborne-disease outbreaks—United States, 1988–1992. *MMWR CDC Surveill Summ.* 1996;45:1–66.

Behari M, Raju GB. Electrophysiological studies in patients with blepharospasm after *botulinum* toxin A therapy. *J Neurol Sci.* 1996;135:74–77.

Beutler AM, Schumacher HR, Jr. Reactive arthritis: is it a useful concept? *Brit J Clin Pract.* 1997;51:169–172.

Bleck T. *Clostridium botulinum.* In: Mandell G, Bennett J, Dolin R, eds. *Principles and Practice of Infectious Diseases.* 5th ed. Vol. 2. New York: Churchill Livingstone, Inc.; 2000:1885–1889.

Bolyard EA, Tablan OC, Williams WW, Pearson ML, Shapiro CN, Deitchman SD. Guideline for infection control in health care personnel, 1998. Atlanta: Centers for Disease Control and Prevention; 1998.

Bond PA. A role for herpes simplex virus in the aetiology of chronic fatigue syndrome and related disorders. *Medical Hypotheses*. 1993;40(5):301–308.

Bonkovsky HL. Therapy of hepatitis C: other options. *Hepatology*. 1997;26:143S–151S.

Brady WM. Controversies in diagnosis and treatment of hepatitis C. Which patients benefit most from therapy? *Postgrad Med*. 1997;102:201–202, 205–207, 211–212.

Braun J, Sieper J. The sacroiliac joint in the spondyloarthropathies. *Current Opinion in Rheumatology*. 1996;8:275–287.

Brindley PJ. Drug resistance to schistosomicides and other antihelminthics of medical significance. *Acta Trop*. 1994;56:213–231.

Burans JP, Sharp T, Wallace M, et al. Threat of hepatitis E virus infection in Somalia during Operation Restore Hope. *Clin Infect Dis*. 1994;18:100–102.

Burmester GR, Daser A, Kamradt T, et al. Immunology of reactive arthritides. *Ann Rev Immunol*. 1995;13:229–250.

Burt FJ, Leman PA, Abbott JC, Swanepoel R. Serodiagnosis of Crimean-Congo haemorrhagic fever. *Epidemiol Infect*. 1994;113:551–562.

Burt FJ, Leman PA, Smith JF, Swanepoel R. The use of a reverse transcription-polymerase chain reaction for the detection of viral nucleic acid in the diagnosis of Crimean-Congo haemorrhagic fever. *J Virol Methods*. 1998;70:129–137.

Butterworth AE, Curry AJ, Dunne DW, et al. Immunity and morbidity in human schistosomiasis mansoni. *Trop Geogr Med*. 1994;46:197–208.

Butterworth AE, Dunne DW, Fulford AJ, Ouma JH, Sturrock RF. Immunity and morbidity in *Schistosoma mansoni* infection: quantitative aspects. *Am J Trop Med Hyg*. 1996;55:109–115.

Cecchine G, et al. A *Review of the Scientific Literature As It Pertains to Gulf War Illnesses*, Vol. 8: *Pesticides*. Santa Monica, Calif.: RAND, MR-1018/8, forthcoming.

Centers for Disease Control and Prevention. Case definitions for public health surveillance. *MMWR*. 1990;39(RR13):43.

Centers for Disease Control and Prevention. Rabies Prevention—United States, 1991 Recommendations of the Advisory Committee on Immunization Practices (ACIP). *MMWR*. 1991;40(RR03):1–19.

Centers for Disease Control and Prevention. Update: management of patients with suspected viral hemorrhagic fever—United States. *JAMA*. 1995;274:374–375.

Centers for Disease Control and Prevention. Control and prevention of meningococcal disease and control and prevention of serogroup C meningo-coccal disease: Evaluation and management of suspected outbreaks. *MMWR*. 1997a;46:13–21.

Centers for Disease Control and Prevention. Malaria Surveillance—United States, 1997, MMWR. 1997b,46(SS-5);1–16.

Centers for Disease Control and Prevention. Botulism in the United States, 1899–1996. Handbook for Epidemiologists, Clinicians, and Laboratory Workers. Atlanta, GA: 1998.

Centers for Disease Control and Prevention. Biological and chemical terrorism: Strategic plan for preparedness and response. Recommendations of the CDC Strategic Planning Workgroup. *MMWR*. 2000;49(RR04):1–14.

Charoenratanakul S. Tropical infection and the lung. *Monaldi Arch Chest Dis*. 1997;52:376–379.

Cheever AW. Differential regulation of granuloma size and hepatic fibrosis in schistosome infections. *Mem Inst Oswaldo Cruz*. 1997;92:689–692.

Choppa PC, Vojdani A, Tagle C, Andrin R, Magtoto L. Multiplex PCR for the detection of *Mycoplasma fermentans*, *M. hominis* and *M. penetrans* in cell cultures and blood samples of patients with chronic fatigue syndrome. *Molecular and Cellular Probes*. 1998;12(5):301–308.

Chung IK, Armstrong TC, Patterson JL. Identification of a short viral transcript in Leishmania RNA virus-infected cells. *Virology*. 1994;198:552–556.

Co MC, Jr. *Mycobacterium tuberculosis* in persons infected with the human immunodeficiency virus. *Am J Crit Care*. 1994;3:389–397.

Cole B, Ward J. *Mycoplasmas* as arthritogenic agents. In: Tully J, Whitcomb R, eds. *Human and Animal Mycoplasmas*. New York, NY: Academic Press; 1979:367–398.

Connor SJ, Thomson MC, Flasse SP, Perryman AH. Environmental information systems in malaria risk mapping and epidemic forecasting. *Disasters*. 1998;22:39–56.

Cook GC. *Entamoeba histolytica* and *Giardia lamblia* infections: current diag-nostic strategies. *Parasite*. 1995;2:107–112.

Cooper CW. Risk factors in transmission of brucellosis from animals to humans in Saudi Arabia. *Trans R Soc Trop Med Hyg*. 1992;86:206–209.

Cope SE, Schultz GW, Richards AL, et al. Assessment of arthropod vectors of infectious diseases in areas of U.S. troop deployment in the Persian Gulf. *Am J Trop Med Hyg.* 1996;54:49–53.

Corbel MJ. Brucellosis: an overview. *Emerg Infect Dis.* 1997;3:213–221.

Corey L. Rabies, rhabdoviruses, and marburg-like agents. In: Wilson J, Braunwald E, Isselbacher K, et al., eds. *Principles of Internal Medicine.* 12th ed. New York: McGraw Hill, Inc.; 1991:720–725.

Cross ER, Hyams KC. The potential effect of global warming on the geographic and seasonal distribution of *Phlebotomus papatasi* in southwest Asia. *Environ Health Perspect.* 1996;104:724–727.

Cross ER, Newcomb WW, Tucker CJ. Use of weather data and remote sensing to predict the geographic and seasonal distribution of *Phlebotomus papatasi* in southwest Asia. *Am J Trop Med Hyg.* 1996;54:530–536.

Daley CL. Current issues in the pathogenesis and management of HIV-related tuberculosis. *AIDS Clin Rev.* 1997:289–321.

Damen M, Bresters D. Hepatitis C treatment. *Curr Stud Hematol Blood Transfus.* 1998:181–207.

Defense Science Board. Report of the Defense Science Board Task Force on Persian Gulf War Health Effects. Washington, D.C.: Office of the Under Secretary of Defense for Acquisition and Technology; 1994.

Department of Defense, Comprehensive Clinical Evaluation Program. CCEP Report on 18,598 Participants. Washington, D.C.;1996.

Dillon DC, Day CH, Whittle JA, Magill AJ, Reed SG. Characterization of a *Leishmania tropica* antigen that detects immune responses in Desert Storm viscerotropic leishmaniasis patients. *Proc Natl Acad Sci U S A.* 1995;92:7981–7985.

du Plessis JP, Govendrageloo K, Levin SE. Right-sided endocarditis due to *Salmonella typhi. Pediatr Cardiol.* 1997;18:443–444.

Dubois P, Pereira da Silva L. Towards a vaccine against asexual blood stage infection by *Plasmodium falciparum. Res Immunol.* 1995;146:263–275.

Duerksen S. Infection may hold clue to Gulf ills: bacteria being found in many ailing vets. *San Diego Union Tribune.* March 22, 2000.

Ebringer A, Wilson C. HLA molecules, bacteria and autoimmunity. *J Med Microbiol.* 2000;49:305–311.

el-Hazmi MA. Hepatitis A antibodies: prevalence in Saudi Arabia. *J Trop Med Hyg.* 1989a;92:427–430.

el-Hazmi MA. Hepatitis B virus in Saudi Arabia. *J Trop Med Hyg*. 1989b;92:56–61.

Elliott DE. Schistosomiasis. Pathophysiology, diagnosis, and treatment. *Gastroenterol Clin North Am*. 1996;25:599–625.

Esper GJ, Charles PD, Davis TL, Robertson D. Adult-onset focal dystonias: presentation and treatment. *Tenn Med*. 1997;90:18–20.

Everhart JE, Stolar M, Hoofnagle JH. Management of hepatitis C: a national survey of gastroenterologists and hepatologists. *Hepatology*. 1997;26:78S–82S.

Facer CA, Tanner M. Clinical trials of malaria vaccines: progress and prospects. *Adv Parasitol*. 1997;39:1–68.

Fishbein D, Bernard K. Rabies virus. In: Mandell G, Bennett J, Dolin R, eds. *Principles and Practice of Infectious Diseases*. Vol. 2. 5th ed. New York: Churchill Livingstone, Inc.; 2000:1527–1543.

Fisher-Hoch SP, Khan JA, Rehman S, Mirza S, Khurshid M, McCormick JB. Crimean-Congo haemorrhagic fever treated with oral ribavirin. *Lancet*. 1995;346:472–475.

Food and Drug Administration, CBER. Fact sheet re: Potential mycoplasma contamination and anthrax and *botulinum* toxoid vaccines. 1996.

Fredericks DN, Relman DA. Sequence-based identification of microbial pathogens: a reconsideration of Koch's postulates. *Clin Microbiol Rev*. 1996;9:18–33.

Frost F, Craun G, Calderon R. Increasing hospitalization and death possibly due to *Clostridium difficile* diarrheal disease. *Emerg Infect Dis*. 1998;4:619–625.

Fujihara T, Nagai Y, Kubo T, Seki S, Satake K. Amebic liver abscess. *J Gastroenterol*. 1996;31:659–663.

Fukuda K, Nisenbaum R, Stewart G, et al. Chronic multisymptom illness affecting Air Force veterans of the Gulf War. *JAMA*. 1998;280:981–988.

Fule RP, Chidgupkar J. *Salmonella typhi* septic arthritis of elbow—a case report. *Indian J Med Sci*. 1994;48:161–162.

Gad El-Rab MO, Kambal AM. Evaluation of a *Brucella* enzyme immunoassay test (ELISA) in comparison with bacteriological culture and agglutination. *J Infect*. 1998;36:197–201.

Gaviria-Ruiz MM, Cardona-Castro NM. Evaluation and comparison of different blood culture techniques for bacteriological isolation of *Salmonella typhi* and *Brucella abortus*. *J Clin Microbiol*. 1995;33:868–871.

Golomb B. *A Review of the Scientific Literature As It Pertains to Gulf War Illnesses,* Vol. 2: *Pyridostigmine Bromide.* Santa Monica, Calif.: RAND, MR-1018/2, 1999.

Golomb B. *A Review of the Scientific Literature As It Pertains to Gulf War Illnesses,* Vol. 3: *Immunizations.* Santa Monica, Calif.: RAND, MR-1018/3, forthcoming.

Gonzalez-Ruiz A, Haque R, Rehman T, et al. Diagnosis of amebic dysentery by detection of *Entamoeba histolytica* fecal antigen by an invasive strain-specific, monoclonal antibody-based enzyme-linked immunosorbent assay. *J Clin Microbiol.* 1994;32:964–970.

Greenwood BM. What's new in malaria control? *Ann Trop Med Parasitol.* 1997;91:523–531.

Gubler DJ, Clark GG. Dengue/dengue hemorrhagic fever: the emergence of a global problem. *Emerg Infect Dis.* 1995;1:55–57.

Gupta S, Vayuvegula B. A comprehensive immunological analysis in chronic fatigue syndrome. *Scan. J. Immunol.* 1991;33(3):319–327.

Hagan P. Immunity and morbidity in infection due to *Schistosoma haematobium. Am J Trop Med Hyg.* 1996;55:116–120.

Haier J, et al. Detection of mycoplasma antigens in blood of patients with rheumatoid arthritis. *Rheumatology.* 1999;38(6):504–509.

Haque R, Ali IK, Akther S, Petri WA, Jr. Comparison of PCR, isoenzyme analysis, and antigen detection for diagnosis of *Entamoeba histolytica* infection. *J Clin Microbiol.* 1998;36:449–452.

Hardegree C, Novak J, Chandler D, Malkin B, Nightingale S. Conference Call with FDA Vaccine personnel. Food and Drug Administration; 1997.

Hasan JA, Huq A, Tamplin ML, Siebeling RJ, Colwell RR. A novel kit for rapid detection of *Vibrio cholerae* O1. *J Clin Microbiol.* 1994;32:249–252.

Hayashi N, Takehara T, Kamada T. In vivo transfection of rat liver with hepatitis C virus cationic liposome-mediated gene delivery. *Princess Takamatsu Symp.* 1995;25:143–149.

Hedriana HL, Mitchell JL, Williams SB. *Salmonella typhi* chorioamnionitis in a human immunodeficiency virus-infected pregnant woman. A case report. *J Reprod Med.* 1995;40:157–159.

Heintges T, Wands JR. Hepatitis C virus: epidemiology and transmission. *Hepatology.* 1997;26:521–526.

Helling-Giese G, Kjetland EF, Gundersen SG, et al. Schistosomiasis in women: manifestations in the upper reproductive tract. *Acta Trop.* 1996;62:225–238.

Helmick C. The epidemiology of human rabies postexposure prophylaxis, 1980–1981. *JAMA*. 1983;250:1990–1996.

Hewage UC, Kamaladasa AI, Amarasinghe AK, Amarasekera N. *Salmonella typhi* endocarditis. *Ceylon Med J*. 1994;39:43–44.

Hill DR. *Giardia lamblia*. In: Mandell GL, Bennett JE, Dolin R, eds. *Principles and Practice of Infectious Diseases*. Vol. 2. 5th ed. New York: Churchill Livingstone, Inc.; 2000:2487–2493.

Hone DM, Harris AM, Levine MM. Adaptive acid tolerance response by *Salmonella typhi* and candidate live oral typhoid vaccine strains. *Vaccine*. 1994;12:895–898.

Hoofnagle JH, di Bisceglie AM. The treatment of chronic viral hepatitis. *N Engl J Med*. 1997;336:347–356.

Hoofnagle JH. Hepatitis C: the clinical spectrum of disease. *Hepatology*. 1997;26:15S–20S.

Hoshino K, Yamasaki S, Mukhopadhyay AK, et al. Development and evaluation of a multiplex PCR assay for rapid detection of toxigenic *Vibrio cholerae* O1 and O139. *FEMS Immunol Med Microbiol*. 1998;20:201–207.

Huang W, See D, Tilles J. The prevalence of *Mycoplasma Incognitus* in normal control or patients with AIDS or the chronic fatigue syndrome (paper presented at the 35th Annual Meeting of the Infectious Diseases Society of America). *Journal of Clinical Infectious Diseases*. 1997;25(2):484.

Hyams KC, Bourgeois AL, Merrell BR, et al. Diarrheal disease during Operation Desert Shield. *N Engl J Med*. 1991;325:1423–428.

Hyams KC, Hanson K, Wignall FS, Escamilla J, Oldfield EC, 3rd. The impact of infectious diseases on the health of U.S. troops deployed to the Persian Gulf during operations Desert Shield and Desert Storm. *Clin Infect Dis*. 1995;20:1497–1504.

Hyams KC, Okoth FA, Tukei PM, et al. Epidemiology of hepatitis B in eastern Kenya. *J Med Virol*. 1989;28:106–109.

Inchauspe G. Gene vaccination for hepatitis C. *Springer Semin Immunopathol*. 1997;19:211–221.

Infection with schistosomes (*Schistosoma haematobium, Schistosoma mansoni* and *Schistosoma japonicum*). *IARC Monogr Eval Carcinog Risks Hum*. 1994;61:45–119.

Inoue K, Fujinaga Y, Watanabe T, et al. Molecular composition of *Clostridium botulinum* type A. *Infect Immun*. 1996;64:1589–1594.

Institute of Medicine. Health Consequences of Service During the Persian Gulf War: Recommendations for Research and Information Systems. Washington, D.C.: Committee to Review the Health Consequences of Service During the Persian Gulf War; 1996.

Iowa Persian Gulf Study Group. Self-reported illness and health status among Gulf War veterans. A population-based study. *JAMA*. 1997;277:238–245.

Jean D, Fecteau G, Scott D, Higgins R, Quessy S. *Clostridium botulinum* type C intoxication in feedlot steers ensiled poultry litter. *Can Vet J*. 1995;36:626–628.

Joo JS, Agachan F, Wolff B, Nogueras JJ, Wexner SD. Initial North American experience with *botulinum* toxin type treatment of anismus. *Dis Colon Rectum*. 1996;39:1107–1111.

Joseph SC. A comprehensive clinical evaluation of 20,000 Persian Gulf War veterans. Comprehensive Clinical Evaluation Program Evaluation Team. *Mil Med*. 1997;162:149–155.

Kain KC, Keystone JS. Malaria in travelers. Epidemiology, disease, and prevention. *Infect Dis Clin North Am*. 1998;12:267–284.

Karlin S, Campbell AM. Which bacterium is the ancestor of the animal mitochondrial genome? *Proc Natl Acad Sci U S A*. 1994;91:12842–12846.

Kaye D. Brucellosis. In: Wilson JD, Braunwald E, Isselbacher KJ, et al., eds. *Principles of Internal Medicine*. 12th ed. New York: McGraw-Hill, Inc.; 1991:625–626.

Keat A. Reactive arthritis. *Advances in Experimental Medicine and Biology*. 1999;455:201–206.

Keusch GT. Salmonellosis. In: Wilson JD, Braunwald E, Isselbacher KJ, et al., eds. *Principles of Internal Medicine*. 12th ed. New York: McGraw Hill, Inc.; 1991:609–613.

Kitua AY. Field trials of malaria vaccines. *Indian J Med Res*. 1997;106:95–108.

Klugman KP, Koornhof HJ, Robbins JB, Le Cam NN. Immunogenicity, efficacy and serological correlate of protection of *Salmonella typhi* Vi capsular polysaccharide vaccine three years after immunization. *Vaccine*. 1996;14:435–438.

Koff RS. Hepatitis A. *Lancet*. 1998;351:1643–1649.

Kollaritsch H, Que JU, Kunz C, Wiedermann G, Herzog C, Cryz SJ, Jr. Safety and immunogenicity of live oral cholera and typhoid vaccines administered alone or in combination with antimalarial drugs, oral polio vaccine, or yellow fever vaccine. *J Infect Dis*. 1997;175:871–875.

Kreutzer RD, Grogl M, Neva FA, Fryauff DJ, Magill AJ, Aleman-Munoz MM. Identification and genetic comparison of leishmanial parasites causing viscerotropic and cutaneous disease in soldiers returning from Operation Desert Storm. *Am J Trop Med Hyg*. 1993;49:357–363.

Kwiatkowski D, Marsh K. Development of a malaria vaccine. *Lancet*. 1997;350:1696–1701.

Lashof JC, Baldeschwieler J, Caplan AL, et al. Presidential Advisory Committee on Gulf War Veterans' Illnesses: Final Report. Washington, D.C.: U.S. Government Printing Office; 1996.

Lederberg J. Infectious disease as an evolutionary paradigm. *Emerg Infect Dis*. 1997;3:417–423.

Lemon SM. Type A viral hepatitis: epidemiology, diagnosis, and prevention. *Clin Chem*. 1997;43:1494–1499.

Leo YS, Chew SK, Allen DM, Monteiro EH. Malaria: prophylaxis and therapy. *Singapore Med J*. 1994;35:509–511.

Lever W, Schaumburg-Lever G. Diseases caused by protozoa. In: Lever W, Schaumburg-Lever G, eds. *Histopathology of the Skin*. 6th ed. Philadelphia: JB Lippincott Co; 1983:356–359.

Levine MM, Galen J, Barry E, et al. Attenuated *Salmonella* as live oral vaccines against typhoid fever and as live vectors. *J Biotechnol*. 1996;44:193–196.

Lew D. *Bacillus Anthracis* (Anthrax). In: Mandell GL, Bennett JE, Dolin R, eds. *Principles and Practice of Infectious Diseases*. Vol. 2. 5th ed. New York: Churchill Livingstone, Inc.; 2000:1885–1889.

Lisitsyn NA. Representational difference analysis: finding the genomes. *Trends Genet*. 1995;11:303–307.

Lo S. Mycoplasmas and AIDS. In: Maniloff J, McElhaney R, Finch L, Baseman J, eds. *Mycoplasmas: Molecular Biology and Pathogenesis Mycoplasmas and AIDS*. Washington, D.C.: American Society for Microbiology; 1992:525–545.

Locksley R. Leishmaniasis. In: Wilson J, Barunwald E, Isselbacher K, et al., eds. *Harrison's Principles of Internal Medicine*. 12th ed. New York: McGraw-Hill Inc; 1991:789–790.

Lujan HD, Mowatt MR, Nash TE. Mechanisms of *Giardia lamblia* differentiation into cysts. *Microbiol Mol Biol Rev*. 1997;61:294–304.

MacBeth KJ, Patterson JL. Single-site cleavage in the 5'-untranslated region of Leishmaniavirus RNA is mediated by the viral capsid protein. *Proc Natl Acad Sci U S A*. 1995;92:8994–8998.

Magill AJ, Grögl M, Gasser RA, Jr., Sun W, Oster CN. Visceral infection caused by *Leishmania tropica* in veterans of Operation Desert Storm. *N Engl J Med.* 1993;328:1383–1387.

Marshall G, Davis L, Sherbourne C. *A Review of the Scientific Literature As It Pertains to Gulf War Illnesses,* Vol. 4: *Stress.* Santa Monica, Calif.: RAND, MR-1018/4, 1999.

Marty A. *Mycoplasma* Infections. *Uniform Services University of the Health Sciences Department of Pathology Syllabus VI.* Washington, DC: Armed Forces Institute of Pathology; 1993:91–94.

McCarthy MC, Burans JP, Constantine NT, et al. Hepatitis B and HIV in Sudan: a serosurvey for hepatitis B and human immunodeficiency virus antibodies among sexually active heterosexuals. *Am J Trop Med Hyg.* 1989;41:726–731.

McCombie SC. Treatment seeking for malaria: a review of recent research. *Soc Sci Med.* 1996;43:933–945.

McCully R, Barron C, Cheever A. Schistosomiasis. In: Binford C, Connor D, eds. *Pathology of Tropical and Extraordinary Diseases.* Washington, DC: Armed Forces Institute of Pathology; 1976:482–508.

Mefloquine and malaria prophylaxis. *Drug Ther Bull.* 1998;36:20–22.

Mills A. Operational research on the economics of insecticide-treated mosquito nets: lessons of experience. *Ann Trop Med Parasitol.* 1998;92:435–447.

Moehringer J. Gulf War ailment called contagious. *Los Angeles Times.* Los Angeles; 1997:1, 32.

Monath T. Flaviviruses. In: Mandell G, Bennett J, Dolin R, eds. *Principles and Practice of Infectious Diseases.* Vol. 2. 5th ed. New York: Churchill Livingstone, Inc.; 1995:1465–1474.

Morris W, Knauer CM. Cardiopulmonary manifestations of schistosomiasis. *Semin Respir Infect.* 1997;12:159–170.

Moutschen M, Triffaux JM, Demonty J, Legros JJ, Lefebvre PJ. Pathogenic tracks in fatigue syndromes. *Acta Clinica Belgica.* 1994;49(6):274–289.

Murray C, Lopez A. *The Global Burden of Disease: A Comprehensive Assessment of Mortality and Disability from Diseases, Injuries and Risk Factors in 1990 and Projected to 2020.* Geneva: World Health Organization; 1996.

Nash TE. Schistosomiasis. In: Wilson JD, Braunwald E, Isselbacher KJ, et al., eds. *Principles of Internal Medicine.* 12th ed. New York: McGraw Hill, Inc.; 1991:813–817.

Nasralla M, Haier J, Nicolson GL. Multiple mycoplasmal infections detected in blood of patients with chronic fatigue syndrome and/or fibromyalgia syndrome. *Eur J Clin Microbiol & Infect Dis*. 1999;18(12):859–865.

Newcombe J, Cartwright K, Palmer WH, McFadden J. PCR of peripheral blood for diagnosis of meningococcal disease. *J Clin Microbiol*. 1996;34:1637–1640.

Ni H, Knight AI, Cartwright K, Palmer WH, McFadden J. Polymerase chain reaction for diagnosis of meningococcal meningitis. *Lancet*. 1992a;340:1432–1434.

Ni H, Knight AI, Cartwright KA, McFadden JJ. Phylogenetic and epidemiological analysis of *Neisseria meningitidis* using DNA probes. *Epidemiol Infect*. 1992b;109:227–239.

Nicolson G, Nicolson N. Chronic fatigue illnesses associated with service in Operation Desert Storm. Were biological weapons used against our forces in the Gulf War? *Townsend Letter for Doctors and Patients*; 1996:42–48.

Nicolson G, Nicolson N. Written Testimony to Committee on Government Reform and Oversight, Subcommittee on Human Resource and Intergovernmental Relations. *U.S. House of Representatives*. Washington, D.C.; 1997.

Nicolson GL, Bruton DM, Jr, Nicolson NL. Chronic fatigue illness and Operation Desert Storm. *J Occup Environ Med*. 1996;38:14–16.

Nicolson GL, Nicolson NL, Nasralla M. Mycoplasmal infections and fibromyalgia/chronic fatigue illness (Gulf War Illness) associated with deployment to Operation Desert Storm. *International Journal of Medicine*. 1998;1:80–89.

Niklasson B. Sindbis and Sindbis-like viruses. In: Monath T, ed. *The arboviruses: Epidemiology and Ecology*. Boca Raton, FL: CRC Press; 1988:167–176.

Norder H, Lundstrom JO, Kozuch O, Magnius LO. Genetic relatedness of Sindbis virus strains from Europe, Middle East, and Africa. *Virology*. 1996;222:440–445.

Nordstrom DC. Reactive arthritis, diagnosis and treatment: a review. *Acta Orthopaedica Scand*. 1996;67:196–201.

O'Dell JR, Haire CE, Palmer W, et al. Treatment of early rheumatoid arthritis with minocycline or placebo: results of a randomized, double-blind, placebo-controlled trial. *Arthritis Rheum*. 1997;40:842–848.

Offley E. Gulf War illness linked to Iraqi germ weapons: Gene-altered bacterium found in vets' blood. *Seattle Post-Intelligence*. Seattle; 1996:A1, A10.

Oldfield EC 3rd., Wallace M, Hyams K, Yousif A, Lewis D, Bourgeois A. Endemic infectious diseases of the Middle East. *Rev Infectious Dis.* 1991;13(Suppl 3):S199–S217.

Olivieri I, Barozzi L, Padula A, De Matteis M, Pavlica P. Clinical manifestations of seronegative spondyloarthropathies. *Eur J Radiol.* 1998;27 Suppl 1:S3–S6.

Olliaro P, Nevill C, LeBras J, et al. Systematic review of amodiaquine treatment in uncomplicated malaria. *Lancet.* 1996;348:1196–1201.

Oppenheim BA. Antibiotic resistance in *Neisseria meningitidis. Clin Infect Dis.* 1997;24 Suppl 1:S98–S101.

Ortega YR, Adam RD. *Giardia*: overview and update. *Clin Infect Dis.* 1997;25:545–550.

Parrish NM, Dick JD, Bishai WR. Mechanisms of latency in *Mycobacterium tuberculosis. Trends Microbiol.* 1998;6:107–112.

Peltola H. Meningococcal vaccines. Current status and future possibilities. *Drugs.* 1998;55:347–366.

Peters C, Dalrymple J. Alphaviruses. In: Fields B, Knipe D, eds. *Virology.* 2nd ed. New York: Raven Press; 1990:713–761.

Pittella JE. Neuroschistosomiasis. *Brain Pathol.* 1997;7:649–662.

Plorde JJ. Amebiasis. In: Wilson JD, Braunwald E, Isselbacher KJ, et al., eds. *Principles of Internal Medicine.* 12th ed. New York: McGraw Hill, Inc.; 1991a:778–782.

Plorde JJ. Giardiasis. In: Wilson JD, Braunwald E, Isselbacher KJ, et al., eds. *Principles of Internal Medicine.* 12th ed. New York: McGraw Hill, Inc.; 1991b:802–803.

Pollack JD. *Mycoplasma* genes: a case for reflective annotation. *Trends Microbiol.* 1997;5:413–419.

Porter JD, McAdam KP. The re-emergence of tuberculosis. *Ann Rev Public Health.* 1994;15:303–323.

Qadri F, Azim T, Chowdhury A, Hossain J, Sack RB, Albert MJ. Production, characterization, and application of monoclonal antibodies to *Vibrio cholerae* O139 synonym Bengal. *Clin Diagn Lab Immunol.* 1994;1:51–54.

Quin NE. The impact of diseases on military operations in the Persian Gulf. *Mil Med.* 1982;147:728–734.

Rabello A. Acute human schistosomiasis mansoni. *Mem Inst Oswaldo Cruz.* 1995;90:277–280.

Rattan A, Kalia A, Ahmad N. Multidrug-resistant *Mycobacterium tuberculosis*: molecular perspectives. *Emerg Infect Dis.* 1998;4:195–209.

Ravdin JI. Amebiasis. *Clin Infect Dis.* 1995;20:1453–1464.

Rebolleda G, Munoz Negrete FJ. *Botulinum* toxin treatment of Hertwig-Magendie sign. *Eur J Ophthalmol.* 1996;6:217–219.

Reid-Sanden F, Dobbins J, Smith J, Fishbein D. Rabies surveillance, United States during 1989. *J Am Vet Med Assoc.* 1990;197:1571–1583.

Relman DA. Emerging infections and newly-recognised pathogens. *Neth J Med.* 1997;50:216–220.

Ribas J. *Mycoplasma* research at Walter Reed and interactions with Garth and Nancy Nicolson. Washington, D.C.: Walter Reed Army Medical Center; 1996.

Richards A, Hyams K, Merrell B, et al. Medical aspects of Operation Desert Storm. *N Engl J Med.* 1991;325:970.

Richards AL, Hyams KC, Watts DM, Rozmajzl PJ, Woody JN, Merrell BR. Respiratory disease among military personnel in Saudi Arabia during Operation Desert Shield. *Am J Public Health.* 1993;83:1326–1329.

Richards AL, Malone JD, Sheris S, et al. Arbovirus and rickettsial infections among combat troops during Operation Desert Shield/Desert Storm. *J Infect Dis.* 1993;168:1080–1081.

Richman DA. Therapeutic use of *botulinum* toxin type A in cerebral palsy. *Botulinum*-toxin therapy shows promising future. *Rehab Manag.* 1997;10:59–61.

Ruff T. Illness in returned travellers. *Aust Fam Physician.* 1994;23:1711–3, 1715, 1717–1721.

Saez Nieto JA, Vazquez JA. Moderate resistance to penicillin in *Neisseria meningitidis. Microbiologia.* 1997;13:337–342.

Saiz M, Llanos-Cuentas A, Echevarria J, et al. Short report: detection of Leishmaniavirus in human biopsy samples of leishmaniasis from Peru. *Am J Trop Med Hyg.* 1998;58:192–194.

Sampaio C, Ferreira JJ, Pinto AA, Crespo M, Ferro JM, Castro-Caldas A. *Botulinum* toxin type A for the treatment of arm and hand stroke patients. *Clin Rehabil.* 1997;11:3–7.

Sanford J. Arbovirus infections. In: Wilson J, Braunwald E, Iselbacher K, et al., eds. *Principles of Internal Medicine.* 12th ed. New York: McGraw-Hill, Inc.; 1991:725–739.

Schiavo G, Montecucco C. The structure and mode of botulinum and tetanus toxins. In: Rood J, McClane BA, Songer JG, Titball RW, eds. *The Clostridia. Molecular Biology and Pathogenesis.* San Diego: Academic Press; 1997:295–322.

Schumacher DJ, Tien RD, Lane K. Neuroimaging findings in rare amebic infections of the central nervous system. *Am J Neuroradiol.* 1995;16:930–935.

Schwarz TF, Gilch S, Jäger G. Aseptic meningitis caused by sandfly fever virus, serotype Toscana. *Clin Infect Dis.* 1995;21:669–671.

Schwarz TF, Nsanze H, Ameen AM. Clinical features of Crimean-Congo haemorrhagic fever in the United Arab Emirates. *Infection.* 1997;25:364–367.

See D, Tilles J. The prevalence of *Mycoplasma incognitus* in normal controls or patients with AIDS or the chronic fatigue syndrome. *Infectious Diseases Society of America 35th Annual Meeting.* San Francisco, CA; 1997.

Sharp TW, Wallace MR, Hayes CG, et al. Dengue fever in U.S. troops during Operation Restore Hope, Somalia, 1992–1993. *Am J Trop Med Hyg.* 1995;53:89–94.

Shekhar KC. Tropical gastrointestinal disease: hepatosplenic schistosomiasis—pathological, clinical and treatment review. *Singapore Med J.* 1994;35:616–621.

Singh BR, Foley J, Lafontaine C. Physicochemical and immunological characterization of the type E *botulinum* neurotoxin binding protein purified from *clostridium botulinum. J Protein Chem.* 1995;14:7–18.

Sinha P, Ghoshal UC, Choudhuri G, Naik S, Ayyagari A, Naik SR. Does *Entamoeba histolytica* cause irritable bowel syndrome? *Indian J Gastroenterol.* 1997;16:130–133.

Soares IS, Rodrigues MM. Malaria vaccine: roadblocks and possible solutions. *Braz J Med Biol Res.* 1998;31:317–332.

Sood A, Singh G, Kharay AS. Role of *botulinum* toxin in treatment of achalasia cardia. *Indian J Gastroenterol.* 1996;15:97–98.

Strickland GT. Gastrointestinal manifestations of schistosomiasis. *Gut.* 1994;35:1334–1337.

Sudiro TM, Ishiko H, Green S, et al. Rapid diagnosis of dengue viremia by reverse transcriptase- chain reaction using 3'-noncoding region universal primers. *Am J Trop Med Hyg.* 1997;56:424–429.

Tesh RB. The epidemiology of *Phlebotomus* (sandfly) fever. *Isr J Med Sci.* 1989;25:214–217.

Thompson SC. *Giardia lamblia* in children and the child care setting: a review of the literature. *J Paediatr Child Health*. 1994;30:202–209.

Tignor GH, Hanham CA. Ribavirin efficacy in an in vivo model of Crimean-Congo hemorrhagic fever virus (CCHF) infection. *Antiviral Res*. 1993;22:309–325.

Tikriti SK, Hassan FK, Moslih IM, et al. Congo/Crimean haemorrhagic fever in Iraq: a seroepidemiological survey. *J Trop Med Hyg*. 1981;84:117–120.

Townes JM, Cieslak PR, Hatheway CL, et al. An outbreak of type A botulism associated with a commercial cheese sauce. *Ann Intern Med*. 1996;125:558–563.

Unexplained illnesses among Desert Storm veterans. A search for causes, treatment, and cooperation. Persian Gulf Veterans Coordinating Board. *Arch Intern Med*. 1995;155:262–268.

Vaccines against meningococcal meningitis: current status. *Epidemiol Bull*. 1994;15:13–15.

Varela P, Pollevick GD, Rivas M, et al. Direct detection of *Vibrio cholerae* in stool samples. *J Clin Microbiol*. 1994;32:1246–1248.

Vassilenko SM, Vassilev TL, Bozadjiev LG, Bineva IL, Kazarov GZ. Specific intravenous immunoglobulin for Crimean-Congo haemorrhagic fever. *Lancet*. 1990;335:791–792.

Velculescu VE, Zhang L, Vogelstein B, Kinzler KW. Serial analysis of gene expression. *Science*. 1995;270:484–487.

Vojdani A, Choppa PC, Tagle C, Andrin R, Samimi B, Lapp CW. Detection of *Mycoplasma* genus and *Mycoplasma fermentans* by PCR in patients with chronic fatigue syndrome. *Fems Immunol and Med Microbiol*. 1988; 22(4):355–365.

Wahren B, Linde A. Virological and clinical characteristics of human herpesvirus 6. *Scand. J. Infect. Dis.* Suppl. 1991;80:105–109.

Weber JT, Hibbs RG, Jr., Darwish A, et al. A massive outbreak of type E botulism associated with fish in Cairo. *J Infect Dis*. 1993;167:451–454.

White NJ. Assessment of the pharmacodynamic properties of antimalarial drugs in vivo. *Antimicrob Agents Chemother*. 1997;41:1413–1422.

White NJ. Why is it that antimalarial drug treatments do not always work? *Ann Trop Med Parasitol*. 1998;92:449–458.

Wiener SL. Strategies for the prevention of a successful biological attack. *Mil Med*. 1996;161:251–256.

Young EJ. An overview of human brucellosis. *Clin Infect Dis.* 1995;21:283–9; quiz 290.

Young EJ. *Brucella* species. In: Mandell GL, Bennett JE, Dolin R, eds. *Principles and Practice of Infectious Diseases.* Vol. 2. 5th ed. New York: Churchill Livingstone, Inc.; 1995:2053–2060.

Young EJ. Serologic diagnosis of human brucellosis: analysis of 214 cases by agglutination tests and review of the literature. *Rev Infect Dis.* 1991;13:359–372.

Zaat JO, Mank TG, Assendelft WJ. A systematic review on the treatment of giardiasis. *Trop Med Int Health.* 1997;2:63–82.

Zannolli R, Morgese G. Hepatitis B vaccine: current issues. *Ann Pharmacother.* 1997;31:1059–1067.

Zimmerman RK, Ruben FL, Ahwesh ER. Hepatitis B virus infection, hepatitis B vaccine, and hepatitis B immune globulin. *J Fam Pract.* 1997;45:295–315.